SLIMMING DOWN & GROWING UP

SLIMMING DOWN & GROWING UP

NEVA COYLE
AND
MARIE CHAPIAN

BETHANY HOUSE PUBLISHERS
MINNEAPOLIS, MINNESOTA 55438
A Division of Bethany Fellowship, Inc.

Published by Bethany House Publishers
A Division of Bethany Fellowship, Inc.
6820 Auto Club Road, Minneapolis, MN 55438

Printed in the United States of America

Library of Congress Cataloging in Publication Data

Coyle, Neva, 1943–

Slimming down and growing up.

1. Children—Nutrition. 2. Reducing diets.
3. Reducing exercise. 4. Children—Health and hygiene.
I. Chapian, Marie. II. Title.
RJ206.C79 1985 613.2'5'0880544 85–15028
ISBN 0–87123–833–0

All names and characters,
though based on true-life stories,
have been changed.

The Authors

NEVA COYLE, Founder and President of Overeaters Victorious, makes her home in California with her husband and their three children. Educated in California and Minnesota, she attended Rasmussen School of Business and Lakewood Community College and is a graduate of the Berean School of the Bible and Valley Christian University. She is presently working on her master's degree in Christian counseling. Neva has a busy speaking schedule across the country in seminars and media appearances.

MARIE CHAPIAN is well known as an author. Her long list of bestselling books include *Telling Yourself the Truth* and *Why Do I Do What I Don't Want to Do?* with Dr. William Backus, as well as *Love and Be Loved, Fun To Be Fit* and *Free To Be Thin.* Marie is a counselor and holds a Ph.D. in psychology. Her full schedule also includes radio and TV appearances and traveling and speaking throughout the USA and abroad.

Contents

Introduction

Dear Parent:

Your child is about to embark on a thrilling adventure in proving God's Word to be true. *Slimming Down and Growing Up* is a thirty-day program designed to teach scriptural patterns for growing thin, patterns that will lead to a lifetime of freedom from fat.

As your child learns to eat God's way and experience His help, you'll see more accomplished than just weight lost. *Slimming Down and Growing Up* teaches children confidence—confidence in God, and in themselves as His much-loved offspring.

For each of the next thirty days, your child will read a chapter in this book, and respond to the questions or short assignments. On Day Four, he or she will begin a Daily Power Time of talking to God, reading a Scripture verse, and writing what the verse means personally. You can encourage this special time by being sure your child has a Bible translation written in simpler language, like *The Living Bible* or the *New International Version* of the Bible.

We know you are eager to encourage your child in this venture. Read each day's chapter together, if you like. Or work together on the assignments. If your child has a special need, you can even repeat a chapter several times, or go back and reread the entire book. You'll also find ideas especially for you

("Just for Parents") with the special information you'll need to support your child on each step on the way to thinness.

God bless you as you encourage your child toward healthier, thinner and happier living outside the painful and confining walls of fat.

one

Get Ready . . .

Have you ever had someone tell you something so wonderful you could hardly believe it? That's what happened to Bonnie when she learned she could be trim and healthy without starving herself. Bonnie is not the only young person who has heard this good news.

Tim's Discovery

Tim didn't want to ride the bike his grandpa bought him for Christmas. "Kids will laugh at me because I'm so fat," he said. But Tim discovered he didn't have to stay fat if he didn't want to. He heard about *Slimming Down and Growing Up*, and he learned about the right way to grow thin. Today he is lean and strong. Nobody teases him anymore, and he is not only riding his bike, but also learning to do lots of other terrific things he only dreamed of before. This boy who never thought he could play sports found he really liked soccer, and is even going to try out for the junior high team next year!

Tim feels good about what he accomplished, and he was glad he didn't waste any more time staying fat. "The best thing about not being fat anymore," Tim says proudly, "is that I can do the same things other kids do and even be good at doing them."

Terry's Choice

Terry is an eleven-year-old girl who hated being overweight. When her mother joined a *Free To Be Thin* group, Terry begged to go with her. Both Terry and her mom completed every assignment. As they learned how to eat in a way that was good for their bodies, both lost weight.

"I didn't starve on my new eating program," Terry said. "I feel good about myself, and after every meal I am full. I just love all I learned. I thank the Lord for helping me."

Now Terry's eighteen-year-old brother, Bill, wants to start attending *Free To Be Thin* classes so he can lose weight, too.

Success Can Be Yours, Too

Do you want to be thinner than you are? We know you can! You can be successful like Terry, and Tim, and Bonnie. Thousands of adults have gotten thinner through the *Free To Be Thin* program. Now, in this book, you'll find a special way for kids to get thinner, and stronger, and healthier, too.

Slimming Down and Growing Up is a thirty-day program that works. In just a month you'll learn new habits and new ways of thinking that can help you all your life.

You won't go hungry as you follow these principles, and you won't be dieting, either. Instead, you'll be learning how to eat God's way. In this book you'll find lots of help in choosing good foods and learning how delicious less-fattening foods can be.

Read just one chapter each day. You'll find out about other boys and girls who have succeeded in growing thin, and how they did it. In a few days, we'll show you how to begin a "Daily Power Time" when you can write down your thoughts and feelings, and your progress. Every couple of days you'll find pages called "Just for Parents" that will help your family know how to cooperate with you.

Maybe the most important thing you'll learn in this book is discovering God as your friend, and learning how to let Him help you, especially when it comes to eating.

Meet Neva Coyle

Slimming down isn't easy. No one understands better than Neva Coyle, the founder of the *Free To Be Thin* program, and president of Overeaters Victorious. When Neva was twenty-eight years old, she weighed 248 pounds! She had tried everything to lose weight—every diet she could find, and every weight-loss group and clinic, too. Even when she managed to lose weight, she always gained it back again.

Neva hated being fat so much that she even went in the hospital for a dangerous and expensive surgery that was supposed to let her eat all she wanted without gaining weight. After the operation she did lose weight for a while, but soon she was horrified to find herself *gaining* again.

After all these failures, Neva finally turned to God. With His help, she lost 113 pounds, and today is slim, happy and confident. What she learned about losing weight and gaining confidence can work for you, too. Other kids have grown thin and stayed that way with the *Free To Be Thin* principles, and you can join them with *Slimming Down and Growing Up* written just for you!

If you're tired of weighing too much, and you're ready to stop wishing and start doing, we're ready to help. A wonderful, new, *thin* way of life is ahead for you.

two

Letting God Help You

Imagine how wonderful it would be to have your own personal super-power source with you all the time. The Bible says you can! God promises, "*The eyes of the Lord search back and forth across the whole earth, looking for people whose hearts are perfect toward Him*" (2 Chronicles 16:9). God wants to share His amazing power, and He's eager to help those who want Him to.

Sara, the Girl with a Temper

Eleven-year-old Sara had a temper that she allowed to explode whenever she felt angry. Her mother said, "Sara is always throwing a fit about something. She's like a walking time bomb."

But Sara felt she had plenty to be angry about. She was angry at her mother for divorcing her father. She was mad at her brother because she thought her father favored him. She growled about her teachers, and complained they were mean to her.

When Sara was angry, she ate. While she was eating, the food seemed to help her feel better. It tasted good and she liked the feeling of being full. The good feeling didn't last, though, and soon she felt emptier and unhappier than before.

As she put on weight, the kids at school made fun of her, and called her names like "Fatty, Fatty, Two-by-Four" and "Porky." Their teasing only made Sara angrier, and she'd go home to comfort herself . . . by eating.

Getting off this unhappy merry-go-round of anger and eating seemed impossible. But Sara found help for overeating *and* her anger. With God's help, she not only has lost weight, but she has become the contented, happy, friendly girl she wanted to be all along.

The One Who Really Cares

Did you know that God is right beside you now, ready to help you, just as He did Sara? God knows you. He knows your name and where you live. He knows what you love and what you hate. He knows what makes you laugh and cry, and He knows how you feel about your weight.

Better yet, He loves you! It makes no difference whether you have blonde or black hair; green, blue, or brown eyes. He loves you the same whether your stomach is fat or flat, whether your feet are big or small. You please Him if you have braces on your teeth and glasses, and you please Him even if you don't.

You'll never hear Him tease you, or make fun of you, or call you names, because He's on your side. You don't have to be thin to make Him love you, either. He won't care about you any more when you're thin than He does right now. He does want to help you grow thin, but only because He knows being thin will make you feel healthier, stronger, and more confident.

Did you know God cared enough about you to help you get thin and strong? Have you ever asked for His help?

Giving Your O.K.

The Lord needs your permission to begin helping you. He won't force you to receive His help. Have you given your heart to Him? The Lord Jesus Christ, God's Son, proved His love when He died on the cross for you. He took the punishment for every wrong thing you'll ever do when He gave up His life for you. Then He came back to life so you could have power to win over wrong things and problems that get you down, like overeating. He can give you His Spirit, His strength, and His understanding so you can know God as your friend and helper.

The Power of God

The Lord is more powerful than you can imagine. He is more powerful than earthquakes and tornados, and He does many miracles for His children. Many years ago, He made a road right through the Red Sea so Moses and the people of Israel could get safely to the other side. He closed the mouths of hungry lions to protect a man named Daniel when he was thrown into their den. The same God who did these miracles wants to live in your heart and guide your life. Will you say yes to Him? He is knocking at the door of your heart and saying, "May I come in and be your friend?"

How to Say Yes

If you say yes to God, you will become His child. He will forgive you of every wrong you've ever done, and He will help make you strong. When He lives in your heart, He can make you a brand new person as He helps you change day by day.

To make God a part of your life, all you have to do is ask Him. Here is a prayer you can use to invite Him to guide your life:

> Dear Lord Jesus, please come into my life and live in me. I want to be your child and live my life your way. Forgive me for everything I've done wrong. I know as your child, one day I'll go to heaven. Thank you for caring about me. Help me and make me strong. I want you to be in charge of every part of my life, including my eating. In Jesus' name, Amen.

Just for Parents

When Jesus said, "Let the little children come to me," He made it clear that children are not too young to experience the strength of the Lord. God's purpose for all of us is to fit into His plan. He wants young and old alike to know the sublime contentment of obedience to His will. Do you believe your child can become thin to the glory of God? David, you remember, was only a teen-ager when he conquered a giant adults were too afraid to face. Like David, your child can win. He or she can remain faithful to a lifetime eating program which honors God.

Of course, struggles and difficulties are bound to arise. Maybe your child will hit periods of complaining, and you'll hear, "Why me? Why do I have to have this weight problem?" Possibly your child will blame the problem on you, or come up with some other excuse. It's during those times that your faith in God, and in your child, will make a difference.

Losing weight can be a frustrating and seemingly endless task, but that doesn't mean the task is hopeless. After all, walking victoriously with Jesus day by day includes struggle, failure, and repenting. Your child will need reminders that when we overeat, we repent and are forgiven. If we skip spending time with God, we can repent and go on. If we stubbornly refuse to exercise, we repent and God forgives. If we have forsaken what we know to be right about eating, we repent, and with God's forgiveness, we get back on track. We are headed for thinness, and we won't stop until we get there.

It won't be easy for your child to change bad habits, so be ready to help with your cooperation and your prayers. Your gentle encouragement and approval (with no nagging!) can spur your child on to succeed. With Christ's help, your child *can* succeed. Believe it!

three

Talking to God

What if someone asked you what you thought about talking to God? How would you answer?

A girl named Connie told us, "I never talk to God unless it's about something real important like when I am sick or something."

Roger said he talked to God when his dog broke its leg. "I asked God to please help Mitzi. She was a good dog and I cried when I saw her with the broken leg," he said.

"I never talk to God," Sally admitted. "I didn't know He was even there listening."

Do you feel like Sally? Perhaps you didn't know God is with you, caring about how you feel, and that you can tell Him anything. Whatever it is you feel—sad, happy, nervous, afraid, brave—you can always talk to God about it. He wants you to, because talking to Him is the way you make Him part of your life.

God Listens

Do you ever talk to your teacher or some friends, and feel like they didn't hear a word you said? God is not like that. He listens, and is always eager to hear what you have to tell Him. He promises in the Bible, "*You will pray to him, and he will hear you. . .*" (Job 22:27). He also tells us, "*With God everything is possible*" (Mark 10:27). It's possible for God to hear you, and for you to hear what He says, too—even about your eating.

Are You Really Hungry?

Sometimes when you eat, you don't want food at all. Maybe you're eating because you are bored. Or maybe you eat because you're sad or lonely or upset or nervous. During those times, it would be a better idea to have a good talk with God instead of eating, so He can help you with the *real* problem.

Jamie, a twelve-year-old girl from Minnesota, didn't think anyone liked her because she was overweight. She wanted to talk to someone about how she felt, but she didn't feel anyone would understand. When she talked to her mother, she'd just tell Jamie she'd grow out of her fat. But Jamie knew she wasn't growing out of her fat—she was growing fatter!

Jamie told us, "I used to come home from school and plunk down in front of the TV set with a snack. I ate ice cream, cookies, and potato chips. Then I'd drink milk to wash it all down. My mother would just tell me she was glad to see me drinking milk."

The more Jamie ate, the more she wanted to eat. She would stuff herself on junk food until dinnertime, nibble at her dinner, and then eat until it was time for bed.

But one day, Jamie decided to talk to God about her feelings instead of trying to eat them away. "One day I came home from school and instead of sitting down in front of the TV set like I usually did, I told God I was lonesome. I told the Lord how much I wished I had a friend." That talk with God was a good beginning for Jamie on the way to getting thin.

Jill Learns to Be Honest with God

After school every day, thirteen-year-old Jill headed to the restaurant where her mother worked. She was supposed to do her homework as she waited for her mother to get off work so they could go home together, but instead Jill would sit in a booth and eat.

Because Jill's whole family was fat, Jill didn't feel embarrassed about her size when she was younger. Her mother even told her she wasn't fat—just big boned. But as Jill got older, she began to realize that she was always the fattest one in any group of kids. Kids began calling her "Fatso" and other nicknames she hated. The worse she felt the more she ate, and the more she ate the fatter she became.

She tried bringing sweets from the restaurant to school, and for a while that made her popular. But when the other kids went off to play or ride bikes or do anything that required physical energy, Jill was left behind. It was hard for her to walk because the tops of her legs would rub together and become sore. Her back hurt because of the extra weight pulling from her stomach, so the only physical thing she wanted to do was sit!

Finally Jill knew she had to lose weight, even though her parents didn't think there was anything wrong with her size. She knew she was going to need lots of help, so one day in the restaurant, she picked up a napkin and wrote a letter to God. All it said was, "Dear God, Help. Signed, Jill." That little prayer, written on a napkin, started Jill on her way to becoming thin.

Jill and Jamie made the Lord their special friend when they told Him how they really felt. God is very pleased when you ask His help in the things that are important to you. Will you tell God your feelings? You can write your prayers, speak your prayers, sing your prayers or whisper your prayers. Whatever way you choose, God is listening.

Questions to Answer

Be sure you answer each one of these questions. Remember, the Lord is with you.

1. What does praying mean to you? ____________

____

2. Does God hear you when you talk to Him? __________
3. Why does God want to help you grow thin? __________

____

4. We talked about Mark 10:27 earlier in this chapter. Fin-

ish the verse by filling in the missing words: "*. . . with* ______ *everything is* ______________."

A Prayer to Pray

Lord, sometimes I am unhappy because I am fat. Sometimes I think I'll never be thin. Please encourage me and show me you are with me, because with you all things are possible. In Jesus' name, Amen.

four

Get Set . . .

"One day," Jamie recalled, "I had just finished a piece of cake, and I was going to have some cookies. (I was so used to eating all the time that it became more natural for me to eat than just about anything. I never really thought it was bad to eat because it just seemed like the thing to do.)

"But that day, as I reached for those cookies, I heard myself say, *'No, don't eat that. You've had enough.'* I knew it was God speaking to me in a way I could understand. That night, I was so happy because I knew God had told me what to do. And I was even happier because I had obeyed Him."

Jamie isn't the only one God will speak to. You can hear Him, too, if you've decided in advance you are going to listen to what He says, and obey it. God has a plan for how He wants you to eat. When you decide you are going to eat God's way instead of following your old ways, He can make you a success at getting thin and strong. Deciding to eat His way means giving the control of your body to God.

The Bible says, "*I plead with you to give your bodies to God. Let them be a living sacrifice, holy—the kind he can accept. When you think of what he has done for you, is this too much to ask? Don't copy the behavior and customs of this world, but be a new and different person with a fresh newness in all you do and think. Then you will learn from your own experience how his ways will really satisfy you*" (Romans 12:1–2).

When these Bible verses say you shouldn't "copy the behaviors and customs of this world," they're warning you about believing things that aren't true. TV commercials tell you that happiness is gorging on cupcakes, or wolfing down as many french fries as you can hold. They tell you breakfast cereals that have more sugar than cereal are "part of a nutritious breakfast." Ridiculous! Following *these* behaviors haven't made you peppy and happy like the ads promised. They've made you fat and weak.

God is not out to make your life miserable. His ways "will *really* satisfy you." When you are satisfied, you feel full. On the *Slimming Down and Growing Up* eating program, you will not learn how to diet, you will learn how to eat. You're not going to starve or hate eating. Instead, you will find yourself learning to enjoy the foods that make you strong and thin.

With God's help, you know you can be thin. You have learned how to pray and ask God for His guidance. All that's left before you are ready to get thin God's way is to decide you'll do what He says. You'll "*give your body to God*," as the Bible admonishes you to do. On page 175 you'll find a chart telling you what a person your height should weigh. This weight will become your goal, a goal you'll agree on with God.

If you're ready to agree with God that you'll let Him help you to the weight He wants for you, you can pray this prayer:

> Lord Jesus, I'm deciding now to eat your way. I believe you want me to weigh ____ pounds, and I'm choosing to give my body and my eating to you so you can make me the thin, satisfied person you want me to be. Today I choose to obey my way to thinness, with your help.

When you agree to care for your body God's way, God promises you success. You can expect Him to help you to thinness just as He did with Jamie. Even if you stumble or make mistakes on the way, you can expect Him to forgive you and help you get right back on track. Tomorrow we begin working on building the new ways of eating that will get you to your goal. Hooray for you! You're on your way to thinness now!

Starting Your Daily Power Time

Today you will begin a wonderful habit that can stay with you all your life. It's called a *Daily Power Time*.

Your Daily Power Time sheet is a private place for just you and God. Here you will write down your thoughts and feelings. It's also a place for you to write what you want to tell God. Maybe yours will be just a short letter to God, like the one Jill wrote when she put "Help!" on that napkin. Or maybe you will write more, telling God all about your day.

As part of your Daily Power Time, you'll read a special Bible verse. When you write *What today's Scripture verse means to me*, you'll be letting God talk personally to you through His Word, the Bible.

At the end of each Daily Power Time, you'll find words to say out loud. Those words are important because God wants His Word to be "*. . . very close at hand—in your hearts and on your lips—so that you can obey them*" (Deuteronomy 30:14). When you read the Bible, it goes into your heart. When you speak it out loud, it is on your lips. In each Daily Power Time you'll have a chance to put God's Word both places He wants it to be: in your heart and on your lips.

Your Daily Power Time will become as special to you as fattening food used to be. It will help you find just the help you need to become the thin, healthy, strong person you want to be.

Daily Power Time

Scripture Verse for Today:

"*Without God, it is utterly impossible. But with God everything is possible*" (Mark 10:27).

My thoughts today: ________________________________

____

____

____

My special talk with God: __________________________

What today's Scripture verse means to me: ______

To Say Out Loud

With God everything is possible, so with Him helping me I will grow thin. I will succeed because He is my Lord and my friend.

Just for Parents

Your child has just accomplished a feat many adults never do in a lifetime. He or she has set a weight goal, and decided before God to head toward it. Will you pray over your child's goal and ask the Lord how you can help your child learn how to eat and grow thin God's way? You can help your child in the following ways:

- Don't offer food in serving bowls on the table. Let your family ask for seconds. "Won't you have some more. . . ?" is an invitation to overeat.
- Salty foods increase the desire to eat more. Things like potato chips, salted nuts and buttered popcorn are non-stop tummy stuffers.
- Buy a calorie counter. We will be starting to count calories and measure food so you and your child can see just how much is being eaten.
- Give up your charter membership in the Clean Plate Club. If you've been the kind of parent who rewards a clean plate with dessert, reconsider now and simply serve smaller portions. Make dessert an option, not a reward.
- Don't serve dessert if your child is full. Allow him to save it for a snack later.
- Observe if your child turns to food when bored, upset or hurt, angry, etc. Offer other suggestions. "Let's go for a walk and talk," or "Won't you help me with . . ." or "Let's play a game together. . . ." You might want to sit down with your child (*not* in the kitchen) and talk. Make plans for your summer vacation, or talk about happy, up and hopeful things and pray together.

Whatever you do, don't comfort with food. "Here, have a little something to eat. It'll make you feel better" will only make the situation worse. Your child will not get better—only fatter.

five

Go!

Five Ways to Get Thin

If we were to ask you what you ate last Tuesday, could you remember? One thirteen-year-old boy answered, "I can't even remember all the food I ate *yesterday*." If it's hard to remember what you ate yesterday or today, it means you are not paying enough attention to what's going into your mouth. The first way to get thin is to:

1. *Write down what you ate today.*

You can begin to get control of what you eat when you write it down every day. At the beginning of the next chapter, you'll find a chart titled "What I Ate Today." Start now by recording everything you ate today—or yesterday, if you are reading this chapter in the morning. Don't just record what you had at meals, but at snacks, too.

One eleven-year-old girl's "What I Ate Today" list looked like this:

Breakfast:	One slice toast with peanut butter, butter and jelly
	One small glass orange juice
	One glass milk
Snack:	Milkduds
Lunch:	One tuna salad sandwich
	One container milk
	Two chocolate chip cookies

Snack: Bowl of cereal with milk
Dinner: Spaghetti
Two rolls and butter
Peas
One glass milk
Fruit cocktail
Snack: Watermelon

Can you see places this girl could change her eating habits? Your "What I Ate Today" list will help you evaluate yourself, and teach yourself new ways of eating.

2. *Plan your food for tomorrow.*

Plan your snacks and meals ahead of time. Planning means you decide ahead of time to say no to two pieces of pie at dinner. You *plan* to have apple juice instead of a malted milk for a snack. You think ahead so the day doesn't take you by surprise.

Tim plans his daily food in the morning. He chooses what he will eat, so he isn't overwhelmed at meal time. He doesn't want to lose control when he has to face the candy counter or the school lunchroom. Tim explains that as he makes his plan, he imagines himself at mealtime. "I plan for a sandwich and orange juice for lunch, no more, and no less. I imagine myself having a fresh pear for a snack. I *plan* to say no to three rolls at dinner. I plan ahead to have just one roll with very little butter."

Jill, whose mother works in a restaurant, has to especially plan what she'll eat when she gets to the restaurant after school. She thinks about what she'll snack on long in advance so the desire to eat won't be stronger than she can handle. "I plan ahead to have this delicious drink I made up with pineapple juice, ice cubes, half a banana and skim milk. I just love it. Sometimes I plan to have a toasted English muffin or bran muffin, depending on how much I have planned to eat for the rest of the day."

3. *Eat three meals and three snacks each day.*

You don't have to give up snacks to grow thin. You don't

even have to give up desserts. *But you must know what you are eating*. That's why it's so important to record everything you eat, and to write out what you will eat for the day ahead. Plan to eat three meals and three snacks daily.

Don't skip meals. Tim told us how he used to think skipping meals helped him. "When I wanted to lose weight I thought I could do it by not eating. I wouldn't eat breakfast and sometimes I'd skip lunch or dinner. I made up for it the next day, though, by eating nearly everything in sight. I got fatter."

There is no reason to skip your snacks, either, if you plan them. You can choose from the many low-calorie snacks listed on pages 47–48. These snacks will fill you up and give you energy.

Every meal and every snack is important. You can enjoy them if you plan them.

4. *Make God an important part of your program.*

God lives in your body. The Bible says, *"Don't you know that you yourselves are God's temple and that God's Spirit lives in you?"* (1 Corinthians 3:16, NIV). Because you are His temple, He wants to fill you with himself. He can turn gray and gloomy feelings to hope. He can turn impatience to patience. He can turn your desires for the wrong foods to sincere desires for good food that won't make you fat. Include God as an important part of your day.

When Tim wakes up in the morning, he takes out his *Slimming Down and Growing Up* lesson for the day. He says, "I like to read the lesson and have my Daily Power Time in the morning before I start the day because it's like spiritual vitamins. It gives me courage. And I say the 'Out Louds' lots of times a day. They make me feed good."

5. *Include someone else.*

It's good to have someone who encourages you. Hundreds of thousands of adults are on the *Free To Be Thin* program at this moment. They encourage each other, meet together weekly, and pray for each other. Maybe you can find a friend to join you on your *Slimming Down and Growing Up* program, too.

Here's what the Bible says about joining together with other Christians: "Is there any such thing as Christians cheering each other up? Do you love me enough to want to help me? Does it mean anything to you that we are brothers in the Lord, sharing the same Spirit? Are your hearts tender and sympathetic at all? Then make me truly happy by loving each other and agreeing whole heartedly with each other, working together with one heart and mind and purpose" (Philippians 2:1–2).

Tell your family and friends about your decision to become thinner and healthier. Jamie told her family she was tired of being fat, and that she was not going to eat like a fat person anymore. She also told her friends at school about her new eating habits, so when she went to a neighbor's birthday party, it was no surprise that she ate only a small piece of cake and said no to the macaroni salad.

Questions to Answer

1. When I overeat I get ________. (Choose one: (a) cuddly, (b) intelligent, (c) fat)
2. In order to be healthy and thin I will eat ____ meals a day. (Choose one: (a) sixteen, (b) two, (c) three)
3. I will eat ____ snacks a day. (Choose one: (a) twenty-three, (b) none, (c) two)

True or False:

____ Breakfast is not all that important on the *Slimming Down and Growing Up* program.

____ Eating when they're not hungry is one of the traits of overweight people.

____ Stuffing themselves on food when they're alone is a trait of overweight people.

____ Telling others that I've decided to stop being fat is a good thing to do.

Daily Power Time

Scripture Verse for Today:

"Don't you know that you yourselves are God's temple and that God's Spirit lives in you?" (1 Corinthians 3:16, NIV).

My thoughts today: ______________________________

____

____

____

My special talk with God: _________________________

____

____

____

What today's Scripture verse means to me: __________

____

____

____

To Say Out Loud

I am a new and different person. I am learning every day how God's ways are satisfying. I choose to be the person God intended me to be.

Six

A Simple Way to Eat

It's one thing to *want* to lose weight and eat right, but it's another thing to *know what to do*. This chapter will tell you what you need to know to get on the program.

You will be selecting food from the "Food Facts" list, and you will be recording what you eat on your "What I Ate Today" chart. You should make your "What I Ate Today" chart in a spiral notebook in which you will also record your weight once a week (for instance, every Monday).

My weight ______		Date ________
	What I Ate Today	
Breakfast: Snacks:	Lunch:	Supper:

This chart will help you become aware of what you are eating. Also, it will tell you *when* you last ate certain things so you don't fall into the trap of repeating the same foods every day. That's dull and boring!

Adults in *Free To Be Thin* classes must decide on a good

calorie limit for themselves. However, for your program you need only follow the Simple Way to Eat chart found in this chapter; choose from the Food Facts list (pages 35–36), and you will be right on target.

When you measure your food, you don't have to worry about being exact. Simply follow the suggestions in the food facts section. It is more important for you to be *responsible* than to be exact. No one is going to look over your shoulder. If you cheat on your program, you are really only cheating yourself.

The key to good meal planning is to provide yourself with the basic nutrients while staying within your calorie limit—the number of calories your body can use each day. A calorie is a measurement used to indicate the amount of energy furnished by a food. If you don't use the calories in the food you eat for bodily activity, the calories are stored as fat.

Caloric needs vary, but all nutrients are very important throughout life. Because you become less physically active as you grow older, your caloric needs will drop. Your correct weight is the weight at which you *look* and *feel* your best. If you stay looking and feeling your best as you grow older, it means that your caloric intake is adequate.

However, if you do need to lose weight, here are some suggestions for you:

- Eat *smaller* portions of all foods than you have been eating.
- Eat less fat, no fried foods; trim all visible fat off meats.
- Use lowfat milk.
- Substitute fruit for rich pastries and sweets.
- Eat fruits, vegetables, and whole-grain breads or cereals.
- Eat *less* food *more* often; for instance, eat 6 *small* meals a day rather than 3 larger ones. You will be less apt to get hungry and overeat.
- Avoid "crash" diets that may lack some of the nutrients you really need.

The plan here allows you to stay well within your caloric limit. If you choose wisely from the Simple Way to Eat chart, and if you choose to eat a variety of foods, you will automatically stay within your plan. Use the Simple Way to Eat as a guideline and use the list of snacks and fast foods on pages 47 and 48.

If you eat at restaurants occasionally, aim for keeping the meal under 800 calories, and you will be able to stay on your weight program without difficulty. (There are some very handy little calorie dictionaries which you can tuck in your pocket or purse to help you figure out how many calories a certain food item has.)

The Simple Way to Eat

BREAKFAST:

- High Vitamin C fruit
- Protein food (choose one)
  - 2 oz. cottage or pot cheese
  - 1 oz. hard cheese
  - 1 egg
  - 2 oz. cooked or canned fish
  - 8 oz. skimmed milk
- Bread or cereal, whole-grain (choose one)
  - 2 slices whole-grain bread
  - 1½ cups ready to eat cereal
  - ½ cup cooked cereal
- Beverage

LUNCH:

- Protein food (choose one)
  - 2 oz. fish, poultry or lean meat
  - 4 oz. cottage or pot cheese
  - 2 oz. hard cheese
  - 1 egg
  - 2 level tablespoons peanut butter
- Bread—2 slices whole-grain
- Vegetables—raw or cooked, except potato or substitute
- Fruit—1 serving (you may save the fruit from meals for snacks between)
- Beverage

DINNER:

- Protein food (choose one)
  - 6 oz. cooked fish, poultry or lean meat
- Vegetables—cooked and raw
  - High Vitamin A—choose from Food Facts

Potato or substitute from Food Facts
Other vegetables—you may eat responsibly
Fruit—1 serving
Beverage

OTHER DAILY FOODS:

Fat—choose 3 from Food Facts
Milk—2 cups (8 oz. each) skimmed or substitute from Food Facts

Food Facts

LIMIT THESE PROTEIN FOODS:

Lean beef, pork, lamb to 1 pound total per week
Eggs to 6 per week
Hard cheese to 4 oz. per week

HIGH VITAMIN C FRUITS (no sugar added)

1 medium orange	½ medium mango	4 oz. orange/grapefruit juice
½ medium cantaloupe	½ medium grapefruit	8 oz. tomato juice
1 cup strawberries	1 large tangerine	

OTHER FRUITS (no sugar added)

1 medium apple or peach	½ cup pineapple	½ round slice watermelon (1″ × 10″)
	½ cup berries	
1 small banana or pear	2–3 apricots/prunes/plums	½ small honeydew melon
¼ lb. cherries or grapes	2 tablespoons raisins	

HIGH VITAMIN A VEGETABLES

Broccoli	Mustard greens, collards and other leafy greens	Pumpkin
Carrots		Winter squash
Chicory		Watercress
Escarole		

POTATO OR SUBSTITUTE

1 medium potato	½ cup corn or green lima beans, peas	½ cup cooked dry beans, peas, lentils
1 small ear corn		
1 small sweet potato or yam	½ cup cooked brown rice	

FAT

- 1 teaspoon margarine with liquid vegetable oil listed first on label of ingredients
- 1 teaspoon safflower oil
- 1 teaspoon mayonnaise
- 2 teaspoons French dressing
- 1 teaspoon butter

SKIMMED MILK OR SUBSTITUTE

- 1 cup (8 oz.) evaporated skimmed milk.
- 2 cups (8 oz. each) buttermilk
- ⅔ cup non-fat dry milk solids

YOU MAY DRINK:

Water, fresh fruit juices (no sugar added), herb teas, Perrier with lime or lemon

YOU MAY USE:

Salt (sparingly)
Pepper
Herbs
Spices
Lemon/Lime
Horseradish
Vinegar

YOU MAY EAT FREELY:

Asparagus
Collards
Romaine lettuce
Green and wax beans
Cucumber
Spinach
Broccoli
Dandelion greens
Summer squash
Brussel sprouts
Escarole
Swiss chard
Carrots
Kale
Tomato
Cauliflower
Lettuce
Turnip greens
Celery
Mustard Greens
Watercress
Chicory
Parsley

TRY TO AVOID:

- Bacon, fatty meats, sausage
- Cream—sweet and sour
- Gelatin desserts, puddings (both diet and sugar sweetened)
- Butter, margarine (other than described above)
- Cream cheese, nondairy cream substitutes
- Gravies and sauces
- Cakes, cookies, crackers
- French fried potatoes, potato chips
- Honey, jams, jellies, sugar and syrup
- Doughnuts, pastries, pies
- Pizza, popcorn, pretzels and similar snacks
- Ice cream, ices, ice milk, sherbets, frozen yogurt
- Whole milk
- Olives
- Spaghetti, macaroni, noodles
- Muffins, pancakes, waffles
- Soda (both diet and sugar sweetened)
- Yogurt (fruit-flavored)

Let's go over in more detail some of the good food you will be eating:

Meat

Lean meat refers to meat that has had all the excess fat trimmed away.

Some kinds of meats have lots of fat that you cannot trim away. Some of these are hamburger, bacon, and sausage. Here's a good way to get rid of some of that fat: cook them until they are well-done and drain the extra grease onto paper towels. You can even eat bacon if you cook it this way. Remember, cook it crisp and flat. If you cook sausages, prick them with a fork in order to get rid of as much oil as possible.

The meats with the most fats are the ones like bologna, salami, and liverwurst. Their fat content is high and their protein content is low.

Poultry

Poultry includes chicken and turkey and can be baked or roasted. If the skin is crisp, you may eat it. The wings have a lot more fat than protein and are more fattening. A good, low-calorie way to prepare chicken breasts is to remove the skin, brush them with soy sauce or low-calorie salad dressing and then charcoal-broil them. Five to seven minutes on each side is enough to get them done.

Cooking turkey too long is a common cooking error. By the time the dark meat is done correctly the turkey breast is often dry and tasteless. The white meat gets done in a rather short time and, when cooked right, tastes a lot better than the disappointingly dry bird we sometimes eat on holidays. A friend used to think that turkey was supposed to come out that way—so dry that you choke on it, and that's why you have to have the gravy to wash it down! Turkey can be juicy and delicious when cooked for the right amount of time.

Also, when cooking poultry, a meat thermometer is a simple way to take the guesswork out of the length of time. And it works!

Seafood

Seafood, which includes shrimp, lobster, crabmeat, clams, and mussels, is excellent for you—low in calories, but high in protein.

You can always have a scoop of tuna fish salad even mixed with regular mayonnaise.

While we're on the subject, let's talk about the use of mayonnaise. Too many restaurants serve soggy, mayonnaise-ridden fish, egg, or chicken salad. Often, all you can taste is the mayonnaise. Use just enough mayonnaise (or diet mayonnaise) to hold the ingredients in your salads together. Using less mayonnaise, you'll taste the meat or fish a lot more and it won't be as fattening. Our butter rule is the same—a little butter should go a long way. Lemon or vinegar is also very tasty on fish. The more you use, the less mayonnaise you will want.

Eggs

Although eggs have a high level of cholesterol (a type of fat in your blood), they are low-calorie (between 70 and 80 calories each), high-protein, and inexpensive. You can fix them a lot of different ways. You can have them fried or scrambled for breakfast, in egg salad for lunch (light on the mayonnaise, remember), and as omelets for supper.

A lot of kids say, "I'm sick of eggs for breakfast. I can't look at another egg." How about egg salad for breakfast? You may look surprised and say, "Egg salad for breakfast? I never thought of that." It tastes pretty good in the summertime when you have it on a piece of melba toast with a slice of fresh tomato. It makes a delicious breakfast and something a little bit different.

Cheese

Cheese is another good food which can be used many different ways. It's also an excellent source of protein. But beware of American cheese and processed cheese foods—and spreads, which are carbohydrate (sugars and starches) solids flavored with cheese. Hard cheese has very little carbohydrate in it because it is made from the curd of the milk, and the milk sugar goes into the liquid portion called whey.

Cheese adds to the flavors of many foods. It's good in scrambled eggs; great when melted on top of vegetables; and, of course, we know and love it in a cheeseburger. In fact, many kids get hooked on cheeseburgers before they get hooked on cheese. That's okay—it doesn't matter how you're introduced to cheese as long as you become more adventurous.

A cheese slicer is fun to use. Unsliced cheese keeps fresh a lot longer, and it's fun to slice the thin slices. Press the slicer across the top, bear down, and you will have beautiful thin slivers. You'll be able to try many cheeses and get to like the different flavors.

Have you ever tried rope cheese? It looks like a big braid, and makes a good snack. You untwist it, soak it in skim milk for a few hours to take out the salt, and then shred it. One braid alone will make a big bowl of cheese strands, which you can eat for snacks. It takes a lot of time and is filling, plus it's healthy.

Most people who eat cheese don't eat it alone. They eat it with crackers, bread, or something else. The problem is obviously in the crackers and bread. If you eat cheese without bread or crackers, you won't eat as much. Cheese is one of the foods that you only can eat in small amounts by itself. If you put it on crackers, you'll eat far more than you really should.

Cottage cheese is a favorite with many teens. We like the low-fat variety. The way to eat cottage cheese is plain, or with raw vegetables, or fruit.

Plain cottage cheese is a satisfactory substitute for an egg in the morning and also instead of potatoes at dinner.

Yogurt

When most of us talk about yogurt, we mean the fruit-flavored kind, sweetened with preserves, or the delicious frozen yogurt, plain or topped with fruit. These treats are fattening, and the carbohydrate count is high enough to serve as a whole meal. If you have a large appetite, yogurt treats won't fill you up, and they have too many calories for snacks.

Frozen yogurt is only 140 calories per scoop and OK as part of a meal. However, it is no better for you than frozen custard or soft ice cream. The only difference would be in your taste preference.

A good way to use plain yogurt in your diet is to mix it with vegetables and fresh fruit or as a substitute for sour cream. Some people make a cheesecake using yogurt in place of sour cream. It's delicious.

Yogurt can be used in many different ways such as garnishing soup or creating meat or seafood salads. One tablespoon of yogurt mixed with one tablespoon of mayonnaise gives you a lower-calorie mayonnaise.

Milk

Milk is our main source of calcium, and in the growing stage, we need somewhere between 800 and 1,400 milligrams of calcium a day. (Boys probably need more than girls because their bones are usually bigger.) One quart of whole milk supplies 1,000 milligrams of calcium and 30 to 35 grams of protein.

Skimming the fat off milk removes some of the vitamins and minerals, but these are then added back before pasteurization. (We say skim milk is "fortified.") Skimming also changes the flavor.

If milk is "one of our most precious foods," why can't a diet consist of a quart of regular milk and a vitamin pill with iron? Well, for one reason it's too boring and, for another, would cause intestinal problems in many people. One crash diet, which has gone in and out of popularity over the years, consists of skim milk and bananas. You drink one quart of skim milk and eat six bananas per day. Nobody ever gets sick on that diet because they get sick of the diet before very long!

Drink skim milk as a high-protein snack to curb your appetite. Skim milk has all the nutrition and almost none of the fat. If you have been a whole milk drinker and hate the taste of skim, switch over gradually. Start by mixing whole milk with lowfat milk; then switch to just lowfat milk; finally, switch over to plain skim.

Salads

Young people often avoid salads because they put them in a "not-too-interesting" category. What they consider a salad is usually some limp tomatoes and wilted lettuce. Salads can be really exciting and delicious. If you're a lettuce-and-tomato or just a lettuce person, you're missing out on some great combinations. There are a lot of different vegetables you can use to make a salad more interesting.

Restaurants often have creative ways to put raw vegetables together. Salads with meat and cheese are not always low in calories, but it would take large amounts of other higher-calorie foods to fill you up as well.

Vegetables

Try different kinds of food, especially low-calorie vegetables.

You should leave out corn, peas, and lima beans from your diet, which may break a lot of hearts—well, maybe *some* hearts! If you only like corn or peas, you can probably have small amounts of them, perhaps half a cup per day. During the fresh corn season you can substitute corn for meat in one or two meals per week. This is because the corn season is short! However, go light on the butter.

Check off the vegetables on this list that you plan to eat:

_____ Acorn squash
_____ Asparagus
_____ Bamboo shoots
_____ Bean sprouts
_____ Beets
_____ Bok Choy
_____ Broccoli
_____ Brussels sprouts
_____ Cabbage
_____ Carrots
_____ Cauliflower
_____ Celery
_____ Chick peas
_____ Corn
_____ Dandelion greens
_____ Eggplant
_____ Kidney beans
_____ Lettuce (romaine, iceberg, Bibb, endive, and chicory)
_____ Lima beans
_____ Mushrooms
_____ Okra
_____ Parsnips
_____ Pea pods
_____ Peas

_____ Peppers, green	_____ Squash, yellow
_____ Peppers, red	_____ String beans
_____ Scallions	_____ Tomatoes
_____ Spinach	_____ Turnips
_____ Squash, spaghetti	_____ Zucchini

If you have checked less than half of these, you are missing out on a lot of variety. Also, many of the vegetables that you eat only raw can be eaten cooked, or vice versa. For example, have you ever tried raw string beans or broiled tomatoes?

Fruit

Fruit is a wonderful and delicious natural sugar snack or dessert. Everyone thinks that fruit is not fattening and that you can eat as much as you want. Not true! It's harder to gain weight on fruit, but, remember, it's still a form of sugar. The tendency to overeat occurs too frequently with small pick-up fruits like grapes. Grapes contain only 3 to 4 calories each, but few of us stop at 10 or 20 grapes. The other smaller fruits, like strawberries or blueberries, are fine.

There is a myth that watermelon is fattening, probably because it tastes so sweet. If you took all the water out of watermelon, you would have pure watermelon sugar (which was used during the Civil War). However, since watermelon sugar is diluted by about 300 times its own weight in water, one large slice is a delicious and acceptable treat. One advantage of eating watermelon is that it supplies a lot of fluid, which fills you up.

Dried fruits are good, too, but remember: they have all the calories of regular fruit, without the water. They don't fill you up as much and so you tend to eat more.

Dried fruits are a very nutritious, potassium-rich food. They pack easily in a lunch box and don't have to be refrigerated. The tricky thing to remember is that if you eat too many, they can be fattening. Raisins are delicious and healthy, and if you stop at one snack pack you won't hurt yourself. But if you're going to eat dried fruit, think of it as fresh fruit: 3 raisins are the equivalent of 3 grapes.

As far as canned fruit, all the fiber and most of the water has been cooked out of it. Much of the time, it is soggy and uninteresting. Most canned fruit is packed in sugary syrup.

When you eat canned fruit, you lose out on the good taste, chewing, and satisfaction of hunger which natural fruits provide, and you get more calories. One exception is canned pineapple: one slice is only 39 calories, so it is a fairly safe dessert.

Condiments

Condiments are seasonings that you add to your food to make it taste better. They include catsup, mustard, soy sauce, terriyaki sauce, Worcestershire sauce, steak sauce, chili, and horseradish.

Catsup has a lot of sugar, but since most people use it in small quantities, it's not a problem. One man mysteriously stopped losing weight when he was told he could have catsup. He claimed he was following the diet perfectly, but when quizzed about his use of catsup, he grinned guiltily. "I love catsup," he confessed. "You might say that I put food under my catsup rather than catsup on top of my food."

Needless to say, that is not how to use condiments. They should add to the taste of your food, not replace it. Going overboard even in seasonings can hinder your weight loss.

Onions can be used as a condiment. They contain a considerable amount of sugar, but small amounts are no problem. Add chopped onion to your salad or your hamburger. Onions may be sautéed in a small amount of butter occasionally to dress up a steak.

Mustard can add to the flavor of a number of foods. In small quantities you can even use hot, sweet mustard that contains sugar. It tastes especially good on turkey, hamburger, and shrimp. A combination of mustard and catsup is good on hamburgers. Mustard is excellent mixed with deviled eggs, or as the main flavoring for a vegetable dip (combined with yogurt and diet mayonnaise). This kind of dip is relatively low in calories and does not have to be restricted to party use.

Dill pickles are a marvelous addition to a diet, although high in salt content. Salt helps keep water in your body.

Dill pickles seem to curb your appetite, and when you put something that sour into your mouth, you don't have as much of a craving for sweets. The next time you eat a pickle, think about whether you really want that piece of chocolate. Pickles are low in calories (15 to 25 depending on the size), require a lot of chewing, and most teen-agers enjoy them.

Salt

Go easy on salty foods because salt holds liquid in your body. It makes you thirsty, too. When you're slimming down, salt (or sodium) should be cut down.

Beverages

Why is it important to drink a lot of water on a diet? Because when you diet, you use up a lot of fat and create a lot of waste. The faster you flush the waste products out of your system, the better you will feel. But don't drink ridiculous amounts of water. You can drink 4 glasses of water per day and make up the remainder of your fluid requirements with milk, tomato juice, and diet soda.

Diet soda still raises questions at the moment. As of this writing, diet soda with saccharine is still on the market. Scientists have found a connection between saccharine and bladder cancer in animals, and it may not be around much longer. Under no circumstances should you drink regular soda when trying to lose or maintain weight. Try Perrier with lemon or lime, natural spring water, orange juice, sparkling apple juice, iced herb teas, or tomato juice. Not only is it refreshing, filling, and inexpensive, but is available almost everywhere. If there's nothing else in the vending machine that looks healthy, there is usually a can of tomato juice.

Soup

Soup can be valuable as a temporary filler for you when you come home starving after school. It is important that you choose a soup that is low in calories. Vegetable, chicken, or beef bouillon can be used. There are also certain homemade soups that contain no fat and are good for you. These vegetable soups plus a protein source like cheese, eggs, and a salad give you a satisfying, low-calorie meal.

If you're using a meat-base soup that's homemade, you must refrigerate it overnight and skim off the fat before it is heated and eaten.

If you love soup, eat it as a first course and give up fruit for dessert. While you're not getting the same nutrients, particularly the vitamins, and are getting more salt, it's still a good substitute, calorie-wise.

Hot Dogs

We do not include hot dogs in the protein section because they are not all made the same way. Some brands have large amounts of fat and filler; others are pure meat (Kosher hot dogs are all beef). The difference in calories is great, ranging from 120 to 180.

Many young people adore hot dogs and would rather eat them than most other meats. You may eat two or three a week in place of meat, without the bun.

The problem with these processed meats is that the fat is disguised; most people don't even realize it's there. That plump, juicy look unfortunately comes from the same thing that makes people look "plump and juicy"—fat.

One way to get rid of some of it is to boil processed meats instead of grilling them. You can get an idea of how much fat there is in a product from the little blobs of grease that rise to the top of the water.

We have included a sample of how a typical week might look if you kept on the program. Look it over for menu suggestions and ideas.[1]

---

[1]From the book, *The Woman Doctor's Diet for Teen-age Girls* by Barbara Edelstein, M.D., © 1980 by Prentice Hall, Inc. Published by Prentice Hall, Inc., Englewood Cliffs, N.J.

	Breakfast	Lunch	Supper
Sunday	½ cantaloupe; French toast (2 slices); skim milk	Cold chicken; tossed salad; Italian dressing; blueberries; skim milk	Roast beef; oven-browned potatoes; string beans; cucumber salad
Monday	Orange slices; cereal (1 cup); skim milk	cantaloupe; cottage cheese	Roast turkey; low-calorie cranberry sauce; carrots; salad with cheese dressing; pear
Tuesday	Banana; poached egg; 1 slice toast; skim milk	Tuna salad sandwich (1 slice bread); raw vegetables; skim milk	Hamburger (lean); string beans; cole slaw; apple
Wednesday	Cereal with raisins; skim milk	Ham & cheese sandwich; mustard & pickles; orange	Chicken broth (clear); baked chicken; ½ cup corn; Caesar salad; grapefruit
Thursday	Orange juice; toasted cheese sandwich (1 slice of bread); skim milk	Turkey sandwich with 1 slice of bread, mustard and lettuce; apple	Omelet (3 eggs) with cheese, onions, and peppers; tomatoes and cucumbers; pineapple (fresh or canned)
Friday	Cold cereal with sliced bananas; skim milk	Yogurt with fresh fruit and raisins	Tomato juice; fish or seafood (broiled); baked potato (pat of butter); tossed salad; skim milk shake
Saturday	½ grapefruit; scrambled eggs; crisp bacon; skim milk	Chef's salad with cheese, roast beef, Italian dressing; unbuttered popcorn	Steak; asparagus; tomato & lettuce salad; diet gelatin with fresh fruit; skim milk

Low Calorie Snacks

FOOD GROUP	SNACKS	MAJOR NUTRIENT
Milk	* 1 cup skim or cultured buttermilk	Vitamin D
	** 1 cup 2% milk	Vitamin A
	** 1 cup unflavored yogurt	Calcium
	** ½ cup fruit flavored yogurt	
	** 1 oz. Cheddar cheese	Phosphorus
	* 1 oz. Mozzarella (part-skim milk)	B Vitamins
Meat	** 1 Tbsp. peanuts	Protein
	* 1 egg, hard-cooked or deviled	Vitamin A
	*** 1 frankfurter	Iron
	* 1 oz. roast, lean beef, ham, turkey, chicken	B Vitamins
Fruit and Vegetable	* 2 fruit-sicle cubes (freeze unsweetened fruit juice in ice cube trays)	Vitamins A & C
	* ½ cup serving any of the following unsweetened juices: apple, grape, orange, pineapple	
	* Tomato juice—1 cup	
	* Fresh fruit cubes—½ cup	
	* Fresh vegetables cut into cubes or sticks (Try raw broccoli, zucchini or turnip with vegetable dips)	
Grain	* 1 slice whole wheat or enriched white bread	B Vitamins
	* 1 cup dry unsweetened cereal (combine several varieties for interest)	Iron
	* Graham crackers (2–2½" squares)	
	* Soda crackers (4 crackers)	
Miscellaneous Snacks and Combinations	** Cheese pizza, ⅛ of 12" diameter pizza	Protein
	** 1 stalk celery stuffed with cheese	Calcium
	* Vegetables with dip	
	* Crackers with dip	

Snacks to Avoid	Candy, candy bars, carmel corn, pie, cookies, donuts, sweet rolls, cake, honey, syrup, jams, jellies, sugar sweetened fruit drinks, frozen sugar sweetened fruit ices, marshmellows, sugar in tea or coffee	Calories Insignificant amounts of other nutrients unless fortified

* 1 serving contains less than 100 calories
** 1 serving contains 100–150 calories
*** 1 serving contains 150–200 calories

You are eating to be good to your body, and not to gain any more weight. That's why you need to consume less calories. All food has calories. A piece of chocolate cake may have as many as 450 calories that don't do your body much good. A juicy red apple has only sixty-one calories, and it is vitamin-packed. Your body wants healthy meals and snacks because it wants to run well, be strong, and have energy.

A candy bar doesn't fill you up, doesn't give you energy, but is loaded with calories. A four-ounce bar of Hershey's chocolate has 623 calories. A sweet, juicy orange has seventy-three calories. How many oranges could you eat before you ate as many calories as are in that one chocolate bar?

Just for Parents

God does not love us more because we're thin rather than fat, but God does love obedience. As you help your child to grow thin, you are supporting a decision to obey the Lord. What a wonderful gift to give your child!

Your child needs to eat correctly to be the right weight. Most overweight people have little realistic understanding for what they are eating, or how much. They only know they eat too much. Most overeating takes place when there is no clear eating plan. That's why we've encouraged your child to begin daily writing down what he or she *will* eat, and then what was actually eaten.

You can make an enormous difference in how successful your child is in planning daily meals. Read the previous chapter to help choose and prepare healthy, slimming foods. Most families adopt the same patterns of eating. If your child's meals have to be extremely different from the rest of the family's, his eating plan can seem like a punishment. A child cannot be expected to have the strength to accomplish a goal if his parents do not support him, especially in eating. His plate may have more fiber and less fat than the rest of the family, but your overweight child should not be made an odd ball.

Fortunately, *Slimming Down and Growing Up* is not based on a reducing diet, but on the development of sound and healthy eating patterns that will do good for the whole family! The *Free To Be Thin* Cookbook is brimming with exciting ideas and recipes for nonfattening foods the whole family can enjoy, and you may find it a helpful resource.

As you plan the day's food with your child, make decisions together in light of your child's and your family's preferences. And don't cut out all desserts. Instead, count them into your plan. Ask your child whether he prefers a cupcake at lunch or a dish of ice cream after dinner. Or serve the dessert in a lessened amount. You can often take one serving, cut it in half, and have it two different times during the day. Don't forget that there are many *low calorie* desserts you can learn to prepare.

When we ask your child to measure food, don't panic. We aren't asking you to carry around a scale and set of measuring cups in your pocket at all times, but discovering how much a cup of something looks like is valuable information. One woman was shocked when she saw what a half cup of corn looked like on her plate. You can say goodbye to fat when you gain this kind of mastery over what goes into your body and your child's body.

As you plan with your child, you can feel good about yourself contributing in this vitally important way to the health and happiness of one you love.

seven

No Excuses for You!

Have you ever heard kids use any of these excuses for staying fat?

- I was born that way.
- Mom and Dad are fat so I came by it naturally.
- Nobody likes me anyhow, so why should I change?
- I don't want to stop eating the things I like.
- Eating is more fun than anything else.
- I don't know how to lose weight.
- I could never be thin because it would be too hard to do.
- I can't help it. Everything I eat makes me fat.
- My mother cooks fattening foods so I have no choice but to be fat.
- I am different than everyone else. Nobody understands that being fat is not my fault.
- Someday I'll grow out of it. It's just that I have a lot of leftover baby fat.

If you've said any of these things, you don't have to again. You don't need to hide behind excuses for being fat, because you're now on your way to being thin God's way. And God won't ask you to do something that is too hard to do.

He said in His Word, "*Obeying these commandments is not something beyond your strength and reach. . .*" (Deuteronomy 30:11). He is telling you that He won't ever give you something to do that you actually cannot do, no matter how hard it may seem. He won't ask you to climb a mountain barefooted in the cold and He won't ask you to stop eating when food is something He made for you to enjoy.

A Land Waiting for You

You are about to own something new. You're going to possess a new land—a land of fun and freedom from being overweight. God made a promise to His people, the Israelites, many years ago, and it still applies to you today. He said, *"I have commanded you today to love the Lord your God and to follow his paths and to keep his laws . . . so that the Lord your God will bless you in the land you are about to possess"* (Deuteronomy 30:16).

You can take this word as God's promise to you. He wants you to live in a land of freedom and thinness. The only thing He asks of you is that you *obey* His word, *listen* to Him and *allow* Him to help you and guide you.

Bonnie Steps into Her New Land

Bonnie's overweight body made her embarrassed and shy. She feared trying new things, and trying to make new friends because she expected to fail. That's why she clung so tightly to the only two friends she had—Betsy and eating.

When Bonnie first met Betsy, they both enjoyed the same rich, fattening foods—lots of candy and cookies, and second helpings of everything. They would go to Bonnie's house after school to bake cookies, and then eat the whole batch by themselves. Sometimes they would eat a whole box of candy bars between them.

If Betsy stayed home from school or didn't go somewhere with her, Bonnie felt lost and alone. When Betsy did something with another girlfriend, Bonnie was terribly jealous. She worried she'd be left out and that Betsy would get another best friend. Bonnie's only times of happiness were when she could have Betsy all to herself, and when she was eating.

But then Betsy began to change. She no longer wanted to do activities that centered around eating. She talked about joining the girls' volleyball team at school, and wanted to take tennis lessons.

Volleyball? Tennis lessons? Bonnie panicked. She hated exercise, and she had never tried sports because she was afraid she'd look dumb. She usually got out of P.E. class with an excuse from home that she had a back problem or a stomachache, or some other pain.

The change in Betsy made Bonnie take a hard look at herself. Fear of losing Betsy's friendship inspired her to want to lose weight, too. She told her mother, "I want to be like other kids my age. I don't want to be fat and I don't want to be left out." But could she do it?

A New Hope for Bonnie

Bonnie's Sunday school teacher told her many times about God's love. When Bonnie realized God loved her enough to care about her unhappiness, she asked for the Lord's help to lose weight. She read these words from the Bible: "*How we thank God. . . ! It is he who makes us victorious through Jesus Christ our Lord*" (1 Corinthians 15:57).

When Bonnie understood God's promise to her, she realized she could have victory over being fat. Her mother helped her get started by providing nutritious snacks, and offering her other rewards than food for doing well.

Bonnie had taken the first step into the land of thinness God had for her. After following the *Slimming Down and Growing Up* program, Bonnie is now living every day strong and thin. She doesn't need excuses anymore for being fat, because she let God help her learn to eat His way.

A Food and Feelings Quiz

1. When you feel angry, do you look for something to eat even if you're not hungry? _____ Yes _____ No

2. If you feel bored, do you go to the refrigerator for something to eat? _____ Yes _____ No

3. When you feel lonely (and we all do sometimes), do you spend more time eating snacks and treats? _____ Yes _____ No

4. When you feel nervous or worried, do you eat something to feel better? _____Yes _____No

5. When you have nothing to do, is eating the first thing you think of? _____Yes _____No

If you answered yes to even one of the above questions, you are expecting the wrong things from food. Food is not a good comforter. Eating can't take pain away.

But you no longer have to eat for these wrong reasons. With Christ's power, you have now stepped into the new land He has given you, where you are free to be thin. Like Bonnie, you are on your way to growing strong and thin.

Daily Power Time

Scripture Verse for Today:

"*How we thank God. . . ! It is he who makes us victorious through Jesus Christ our Lord*" (1 Corinthians 15:57).

My thoughts today: ______________________________

____

____

____

My special talk with God: ______________________

____

____

____

What today's Scripture verse means to me: ________

____

____

____

To Say Out Loud

I can develop interest in eating the right way. I won't be discouraged with the time it takes to learn things like what to eat and what not to eat. I can do it!

eight

Five Habits That Will Add Pounds

Her little brother's eyes lit up when he spotted the chocolate bar Sara had just unwrapped. "I want a bite," he begged as Sara bit into the candy bar.

"No!" Sara snapped at him.

"Please . . . just one bite?"

"I said *no*!" And Sara crammed the last half of the candy bar into her mouth before he could ask again. "You're always wanting a bite of what I'm eating," she growled between chews. "Why don't you get your own candy?"

Sara was angry now because she'd had to gulp the candy bar down so quickly. Chocolate was her favorite thing to eat, and she liked to savor it slowly.

"I'll go to the store and get another candy bar," she decided, "but this time I'll eat it on the way home so my little brother won't pester me."

Sara's actions show us two wrong ways of thinking that can be seen in many overweight people.

One: Sara simply loved what she was eating. She ate chocolate as though it was something dear enough to have to guard with her life. She loved it like a treasure, and wanted it all to herself.

Two: Sara was more interested in eating than anything or anyone else. She did not want to be disturbed or interrupted. Even if her brother cried and begged, Sara did not really care.

It was the chocolate she cared most about.

Do you see either of these behaviors in the way you act toward food? Do you *love* your food, and guard against anyone taking it away from you? Do you care about what you're eating more than anything, and hate the idea of sharing it?

If Sara had thought about it, she would have realized that chocolate was no treasure. What had candy bars ever done for her, anyway, except make her fat and miserable and lonely? She forgot that eating chocolate is not nearly as special as being with friends, or doing something she is interested in.

Jill shows us another behavior of overweight kids. One day Jill told her mother, "It seems like every time I get nervous or worried, I eat too much." The habit of overeating when you feel unhappy may be familiar to you. It's important to recognize this habit because it's important to understand those feelings.

If you're like Jill, you may be wanting something in your life that is not there. When you feel restless and unsatisfied, you may think eating will help, but usually it isn't food you really want.

Jill wanted a friend. She felt lonely and left out at school. Instead of taking steps to meet new friends, Jill ate to try to fill an empty spot. But the empty spot wasn't in her stomach. It was in her heart. She wasn't listening to her feelings correctly.

Three: Jill overate because she wanted to be filled with *something*, but it wasn't food she really wanted.

Bonnie shows us another trait of overweight young people. On a typical day she gets up in the morning, dresses, and leaves for school without eating breakfast. When she gets to school she can hear her stomach rumbling, but she waits until milk break to eat. Then she eats cupcakes, potato chips, or whatever she can buy at the lunch counter.

If she sits with girls who don't eat much during lunch, Bonnie will not eat much either because she doesn't want to be embarrassed. Whenever she can, she eats outside on the lawn all by herself so no one can watch how much she puts into her mouth.

Bonnie's real eating begins after school. She starts on the

way home and doesn't stop until she goes to bed. Most of her eating is done alone so no one can see her. Look at Bonnie's behavior:

Four: Bonnie usually skipped breakfast.

Five: Bonnie ate more when she was alone than when she was with others.

Let's look again at these behaviors. If you want to add pounds:

1. Make eating more important to you than it ought to be (*loving* chocolate, like Sara).
2. Don't share, or let anyone interrupt you when you're eating.
3. Eat even when you're not hungry. (Jill had other needs to be fulfilled.)
4. Skip breakfast, and then eat too much during the day.
5. Overeat when you're alone.

How many of these habits are yours? It is very important to know yourself. Which of them will you begin to change today?

Daily Power Time

Scripture Verse for Today:

"Why spend your money on food stuffs that don't give strength? Why pay for groceries that don't do you any good. Come to me with your ears wide open. . . . I am ready to make an everlasting covenant with you, to give you all the unfailing mercies and love that I had for King David" (Isaiah 55:2, 3).

My thoughts today: ______________________________

____

____

____

My special talk with God: __________________________

____

____

What today's Scripture verse means to me: ____________

To Say Out Loud

I can stop to think about why I am eating what I am eating. I choose to listen to God and to receive His unfailing mercies and love. With His help I cannot fail.

Just for Parents

If you haven't yet made friends with vegetables, fresh fruits, and protein, you're refusing help from some of the best allies you can recruit in this struggle against overweight. We call these foods the Fat Fighters.

Most vegetables are so low in calories that digesting them uses up more calories than they have to start with. For example, two stalks of raw celery have ten calories, but it takes twenty-five calories of energy to digest them. You *burn up* fifteen calories just by eating the celery!

Fat-burning fruits and vegetables include apples, green beans, beets, blueberries, broccoli, Brussels sprouts, cabbage, cantaloupe, carrots, cauliflower, cherries, cucumbers, eggplant, grapefruit, grapes, lemons, lettuce, mushrooms, nectarines, onions, oranges, parsnips, pomegranates, raspberries, radishes, spinach, tangarines, strawberries, tomatoes, and watermelon.

These foods not only help burn up body fat, but are rich in vitamins and minerals that form the fat-fighting enzymes.

Another tip: our bodies use more calories digesting fresh fruit, such as oranges, than if we drink only the juice.

Protein is also a fat-fighting food. Protein increases the metabolism so we burn up 130 to 140 calories for each 113 calories of protein we eat.

When you are trying to cut calories, it is a real mistake to skimp on protein. Your child's body needs protein at each meal to keep his blood sugar level high and to prevent hunger and overeating. Protein is essential to repair tissues and help wounds heal. Healthy skin, hair, nails, vital body chemicals, blood and all organs depend on protein.

Meat, fish, poultry, eggs, low-fat cheese, milk and yogurt are all good sources of complete protein. You can also get protein from beans, lentils, seeds, nuts, whole-grain cereals and breads, and gelatin, though these need to be combined carefully to get the high-quality protein that meat and dairy sources provide.

When you cook for your child, remember that some protein

sources are higher in calories than others. Three ounces of broiled chicken has twenty grams of protein, and so does a cup of cooked split peas. But the chicken has 114 calories, and the peas 290.

One of the biggest enemies of the Fat Fighters? Sugar! You may not think your family eats much sugar, but you may be surprised when you take inventory of your cupboards and refrigerator. There is sugar in catsup, pickles, mayonnaise, Jell-O, most canned fruits, most cereals, and all salad dressings. Sugar can be labeled as "carbohydrates," or a variety of other ways.

Dextrose is a chemical sugar, derived synthetically from starch. It is also called corn sugar.

Fructose is fruit sugar.

Maltose is malt sugar.

Laxtose is milk sugar.

Sucrose is refined sugar (and it is addictive!).

Glucose is a sugar found in fruits and vegetables and is important to your health.

Your child is learning not only what to eat but how to recognize those foods that are of no nutritional value. Many of the *Free To Be Thin* mothers were surprised to find they had much to learn, too. One said, "It was a real shock to me to discover that I was more influenced by advertising and commercials than I was by the truth."[1]

If your family has been addicted to junk food, ask yourself who buys most of these foods for them. The Lord forgives and gives us the ability to introduce new and better ways of eating. *Slowly* wean your family onto a healthy diet. Start by introducing luscious fruit salads, broiled meat, and fresh steamed vegetables. Skip the rich gravies and substitute natural juices.

Try making healthy fruit juices in your blender. For snacks, try raw nuts and seeds, cheese and crackers, yogurt, or fresh fruit. Instead of serving sugar-packed cereals in the morning, feed your family a high-protein breakfast of eggs, cheese, fish,

---

[1]Marie Chapian and Neva Coyle, *Free To Be Thin* (Minneapolis: Bethany House Publishers, 1979), p. 55.

whole-grain bread or toast or a whole-grain cereal with honey.

The Psalmist prayed, "*Bless me with life so that I can continue to obey you. Open my eyes to see wonderful things in your Word. I am but a pilgrim here on earth: how I need a map—and your commands are my chart and guide. I long for your instructions more than I can tell*" (Psalm 119:17–20). As parents, how we need the Lord to instruct us and be our chart and guide as we raise our children and teach them to eat the way God intended. May God bless you with His instruction.

nine

Treats That Don't Mistreat

What happened the last time you did well on your science project? Did you reward yourself by going out for an ice cream sundae? When you cleaned your plate at dinner last night, did you get rewarded with a fat slice of pie? Or maybe two slices?

Life offers lots of opportunities for receiving rewards. Maybe you get rewards for raising your grades, winning at something, cleaning your room faithfully, or doing chores at home. There's no problem in getting rewards. But for overweight kids, rewards can be a problem if they always mean eating.

For doing dishes every night after supper, Bonnie was rewarded with a weekly trip to the chocolate store. When Sara made her bed every morning and babysat her brother, her reward was an allowance, which she spent on candy. To these two overweight girls, their "reward" was really no reward at all!

Carey Discovers a Better Reward

Carey's parents told him that if he raised his grade in history, he could choose a special treat. Carey went to work, and changed his D to a B in a few short weeks.

"Let's celebrate!" his dad said proudly. "What is your treat going to be?"

Carey thought about it. Not long ago, he would have asked to go out for pizza and ice cream. But now God was helping him grow thin. He remembered the promise, "*How we thank God. . . !*

It is he who makes us victorious through Jesus Christ our Lord" (1 Corinthians 15:57).

"Dad, could we go fishing?" Carey asked.

"Absolutely!" his father beamed. "Mom may even want to join us." They made plans to go fishing the following Saturday, and to take a picnic lunch of sandwiches and fruit juice.

Carey did well when he chose a reward that meant *doing* something rather than *eating* something.

Thinking of New Rewards

When you think of a treat, what comes to your mind? Sara knew right away. "When I think of a reward, I think of *money*." "What do you do with the money?" we asked her. "I buy candy," she said.

Sara's reward was not really money. It was eating. What do you think could be a better reward for Sara? How about spending her money on an afternoon at the waterslide?

Here are some rewards that kids who are *slimming down and growing up* have chosen. Can you add to the list?

- going fishing
- going swimming
- going camping
- going to a special movie
- getting to stay up later
- playing video games with Dad or Mom
- having a friend over to stay all night
- getting a permanent
- getting a new record to listen to
- making a long distance call to someone special

Later on in this book we will talk more about rewards, but you can begin to find rewards that you'll enjoy more than fattening food.

The Best Reward

With the Lord as your helper and friend, you are beginning to eat better by nourishing your body instead of just feeding it whatever you want. When you do your daily assignments in this book and talk to God faithfully, you'll find a reward even greater than getting thin. Your personality and your thoughts will be changed to show more confidence and happiness.

God wants to be good to you. In fact, He loves to be good to you. It's hard to do good for someone who doesn't want you to. But you've decided to allow the Lord to live in you and be a part of your life, so He is free to give you His best reward, a happy heart.

Questions to Answer

1. "*There are many who walk along the Christian road who are really enemies of the cross of Christ. Their future is eternal loss, for their god is their appetite: they are proud of what they should be ashamed of; and all they think about is this life here on earth*" (Philippians 3:18–19).

Who is this Scripture verse describing? ________________

Aren't you glad this isn't true of you anymore? Now that you are God's child, your reasons for losing weight are based on the Word of God.

2. Your new motives are described in Philippians 2:13. Fill in the blank:

"________ *is at work within you, helping you* ________ *to obey him, and then helping you* ________ *what he wants.*"

3. God is your partner. He is with you to help you and love you. Who is going to make the necessary changes in your eating habits? ________

4. Who is going to make changes in your attitudes? ______

____

5. Who gives you new motives and purposes? ___________

Daily Power Time

Scripture Verse for Today:

"*How we thank God. . . ! It is he who makes us victorious, through Jesus Christ, our Lord*" (1 Corinthians 15:57).

My thoughts today: ______________________________

My special talk with God:

What today's Scripture verse means to me:

To Say Out Loud

I will thank God no matter what. He promised me victory and I know He keeps His promises. I am His child and He is guiding me and helping me to grow thin and be the person He wants me to be.

ten

Why Are You Fat?

Sara was sobbing into her pillow when her mother found her. "Did something happen at school today, Sara?" her mother asked gently.

"It wasn't at school," Sara said between sobs. "It was after school. A lady was walking with her kids and she pointed at me and told them, 'See, *that's* why I don't want you eating candy!' "

Sara's mother caught her breath. "Why would she say that?"

Sara's sobs changed to anger. "Oh, Mother, can't you see for yourself? I'm *fat*. Everybody laughs at me. They make fun of me."

"You're not fat, Sara," her mother protested. "You're just pleasantly plump. It's healthier to be a little on the plump side."

Ostriches Come in All Sizes

Ostriches have a most unusual way of dealing with things they don't like. Instead of facing trouble, they stick their heads in the sand, and hope that if they ignore their problems, they will go away.

Sara's mother was like an ostrich. She believed that as long as she said Sara was only "a little on the plump side," everything would be fine. But Sara wasn't "pleasantly plump." She was *fat*. Pretending Sara wasn't fat may have helped her mother feel better, but it didn't keep a lady on the street, and the kids at school from making fun of Sara.

Adults aren't the only ones who act like ostriches, though. Kids can, too. Have you ever asked, "Why me? Why do *I* have to be the one who's fat? Other kids can eat all they want and never gain, but not me"? It's like an alien from another planet sneaked into your room one night and zapped your body full of fat while you weren't looking.

Those moans of "Why me?" and "Poor me!" are fine for ostriches who don't want their lives to change, but ostriches can never be free-to-be-thin kids. Young people who are growing thin God's way have courage and power to face truth, and to find out the real causes of their extra weight, because they know God is going to make them thin and strong.

So, Why Do People Get Fat?

Some people gain weight because they're sick. Something is wrong with their bodies, and they need medical help. However, most overweight people who wonder if they are sick will hear their doctor say, "There's nothing wrong with your body. You're perfectly healthy . . . except you need to lose some weight!"

If you haven't had a physical examination for a long time, you might want to ask your parents about getting you a check-up, to be sure everything is in good working order.

Very few people are fat because something is wrong with their body. Almost all overweight young people (and adults!) get fat three ways.

First, *they eat the wrong things*. When Carey's mother took him for a medical check-up, the doctor said that Carey was anemic. That means his blood wasn't as healthy as it should be. "Anemia is caused by poor nutrition," the doctor told Carey's mother.

"How could that be?" his mother asked. "Carey eats like a horse. He eats *everything*."

"He may eat a lot," the doctor answered her, "but he's not eating enough of the right things to stay healthy."

As you follow this weight-loss program, you may find you can still eat as much as your friends do. You may not always eat all the same *kinds* of food they do, though. You will learn which foods you can eat lots of and which foods you ought to eat less of to get thin *and* stay healthy.

The second way some people get fat is *they don't exercise*. More food goes into their bodies than they need, so the extra food is stored as fat. Instead of biking to the park on a sunny afternoon, they park themselves in front of the TV with a bag of chips.

Another way people get fat is to *eat when they're not hungry*. They eat to reward themselves, or keep from feeling bored, or a hundred other reasons that have nothing to do with their body's need for food.

It comes down to this. Your body requires a certain amount of food energy (calories) to keep it going. If you are eating more than your body needs, you are putting more into it than God intended it to hold. That's what makes you overweight. If you are eating unhealthy food, you are filling your stomach while you cheat your body of what it needs to be strong and healthy.

Sometimes it's hard to say, "I am fat because I eat too much of the wrong kinds of foods, and I don't exercise enough." Even adults have a hard time admitting this. It's easy to blame your overweight on your parents, or the cafeteria food, or even on God, for not making your body different. As a free-to-be-thin kid, you're now free to stop blaming others, and complaining about others who eat more than you but are skinny. You can say "I made myself fat" because you know *God* is on your side, and has promised to help you grow thin.

In the days ahead, we'll work on changing in all three ways people get fat. You're already learning which foods are the right ones for you. We'll begin looking for ways to exercise that make burning up extra calories *fun* for you. In your daily assignments, you'll get new understanding of ways to deal with frustration and boredom and anger, so you won't need to eat as much as you did before.

God is at work to change you from the inside out. The Bible says, "*God is at work in you helping you want to obey him, and then helping you do what he wants*" (Philippians 2:13). He's promised to keep on working in you until you're the happy, free, slimmed-down kid He made you to be.

Questions to Answer

The Bible says in Haggai 1:8, " '*Rebuild my temple and I will be pleased with it and appear there in my glory,' says the Lord.*"

And later, God says, *"Don't you know that you yourselves are God's temple and that God's Spirit lives in you?"* (1 Corinthians 3:16, NIV).

1. Who is God's temple? ______________________
2. Who will be pleased as you rebuild God's temple? ______

____

Daily Power Time

Scripture Verse for Today:

"Fear not, for I am with you. Do not be dismayed. I am your God. I will strengthen you; I will help you; I will uphold you with my victorious right hand" (Isaiah 41:10).

My thoughts today: ______________________________

____

____

____

My special talk with God: __________________________

____

____

____

What today's Scripture verse means to me: ____________

____

____

____

To Say Out Loud

My body is God's house. He lives in me and He is giving me strength and courage to build a slimmer, healthier body.

Just for Parents

Have you ever rewarded your child with a rich dessert? Have you ever withheld dessert as a punishment? *Slimming Down and Growing Up* teaches your child to enjoy rewards involving *doing* rather than eating. Food is not a friend, and it should not be a reward. Food is something we eat with care to keep our bodies healthy.

God wants your child to learn to choose those things in life that are good for him or her. We have asked your child to make a list of what he likes to *do*. Perhaps you could go over this list together and help make some of those desires come true.

The Lord constantly rewards us with good things. You may want to reward your child for faithfulness in staying on the *Slimming Down and Growing Up* program. If you do, make your rewards frequent. Don't tell your child you'll buy him a new wardrobe when he loses fifty pounds. That goal is simply too far away. A *daily* reward during these thirty days might be best.

Rewards do not have to be something expensive or time consuming. You can reward your son or daughter by expressing in words your respect and appreciation for the effort given on this program. Words of praise and encouragement are rewarding in themselves. Or you may want to put stars or stickers at the end of each chapter your child completes in this book.

One mother rewarded her child daily by giving points for every one of the sections in each chapter. She gave one point for reading the chapter, one point for answering the questions and Daily Power Time, one point for making a daily food plan, and one point for filling out the exercise sheet. When her child earned ten points, he was allowed to spend them. (Ten points equaled one dollar.) As he lost weight, her child also earned his Christmas shopping money, and both parent and child were gratified.

Though your rewards will be an incentive, your youngster is also learning to reward himself. *Slimming Down and Growing Up* stresses saying words like, "Good for me!" It is a wonderful way for kids to feel about themselves. Self-esteem is a better treat than candy could ever be!

eleven

Your Reasons to Get Thin

"I'm working so hard at losing weight," one girl said to her friend, "because I want the boys to like me, and I know they will when I'm thin."

What do you think of her reason for getting thin? It sounds pretty selfish and vain, doesn't it.

Not every young person who wants to get thin has wrong reasons, though. Carey wanted to be thin to please the Lord. He knew he was not being good to his body when he made it carry all that extra weight. He knew God wanted him to be good to his body, and Carey's desire was to obey the Lord. That's a great reason for getting thin!

Do you know what pleases the Lord? Is it just to be thin? No. Thin people are not better than fat people. Fat doesn't make a person bad. It's not thinness that pleases God . . . it's obedience.

If you have been eating too much, God knows you aren't doing what is best for you. He wants to show you lovingly how to eat what will do you good. When you choose to listen to Him, you are obeying, and your choice to obey Him brings Him great pleasure. Besides pleasing Him, your obedience will also result in your getting thin.

"So our aim is to please him always in everything we do. . ." (2 Corinthians 5:9).

Obedience is not uncool, no matter what other kids say.

When Jesus came to earth, He did not do anything He pleased. He came here and obeyed His heavenly Father. He became our example, showing us how to obey God and have the right reasons for what we do.

Your motives for getting rid of fat don't have to be selfish. Your reasons can be based on the Word of God. Will you say this out loud now?

I choose to be thinner for the glory of the Lord and to please Him. God knows me better than I know myself, and I choose to be obedient to Him and His Word.

Because you want to please the Lord, some wonderful things are true about you that weren't true before.

- You are in control over what goes into your mouth.
- You can be free from stuffing yourself and overeating.
- You use food. Food does not use you.
- You use calories. Calories do not use you.
- Your needs and desires will be fulfilled through the Lord Jesus Christ who loves you and knows you.

I'll Do It with a Smile!

As soon as Bonnie and Betsy decided to stop off at Jerry's Ice Cream Shop after school, Bonnie's mouth started watering. The thought of her favorite dessert, a banana split loaded with nuts and whipped cream, made the daily food plan she'd written that morning seem very far away. "Forget about the plan," she told herself. "Who can resist a banana split?"

But when Betsy sat down in the booth, she was quiet for a minute. "I don't really want a big sundae, Bonnie," she said. "Maybe I'll just have a small cone instead."

Bonnie scowled at her. "I don't want a cone. I want a banana split."

Betsy shrugged. "Go ahead and have one. I'm getting a cone, and I'll eat it on the way home."

Bonnie felt cheated. First Betsy had started liking sports, and now she decided not to give in to an ice cream binge like they always used to. Betsy was changing so much, and Bonnie didn't like it one bit. But she knew Betsy was right.

"Okay," Bonnie said reluctantly. "I'll just have a small cone, too. I guess I'm not really hungry anyhow." Both girls ordered single dip cones and left the ice cream shop.

At first Bonnie felt upset, but soon she was glad she hadn't eaten that banana split. She really wanted to stop eating the food that had made her so fat. By the time she got home, she felt good about herself and glad she had not eaten all she wanted to. She ate dinner that night, and skipped the second helpings. When it came time for dessert, she told her mother, "No thanks. I already had my dessert today after school when I ate an ice cream cone."

Bonnie was learning to exercise self-control when she chose against the fattening banana split she hadn't planned to have. Sometimes saying no to something we think is delicious makes us feel cheated. We have obeyed, but not very enthusiastically. The Bible tells us to "*Do everything without complaining or arguing*" (Philippians 2:14, NIV). By the time dinner came around, Bonnie showed self-control again by refusing dessert, but this time she did it without feeling sorry for herself. She did it with a smile, and pleased herself, and the Lord, too.

A Remembering Prayer

Sometimes you need a special prayer to help you remember that you've begun a new life as a person who no longer stuffs yourself full of food that keeps you fat. Will you pray this prayer out loud? Use it, too, whenever you need special encouragement.

> Dear Lord Jesus, help me to remember that overeating won't help me if I feel depressed. Help me to remember that overeating won't help me if I feel angry or frustrated. Help me to remember that overeating is not the way to celebrate something special. Help me to remember that overeating will not make me feel good. Help me, Lord Jesus, to discover new things to do instead of overeating. Thank you for helping me, and caring about me. Amen.

Questions to Answer

1. *"Our aim is to ________ him always in everything we do"* (2 Corinthians 5:9).

2. Deuteronomy 26:16 says, *"You must wholeheartedly obey all of these commandments . . . the Lord is giving you this day."* From this Scripture, what pleases the Lord? ________

____

3. What are your reasons for losing weight? ________

____

Daily Power Time

When Bonnie said no to the banana split, she was learning to accept a new way of eating. It was a first step for her toward saying no to herself and yes to God. What would you have done? Can you say no to yourself? Can you say, "Not now—later" when you are offered something gooey and fattening?

Scripture Verse for Today:

"Do everything without complaining or arguing" (Philippians 2:14, NIV).

My thoughts today: ________

____

____

____

My special talk with God: ________

____

____

____

What today's Scripture verse means to me: ________

____

To Say Out Loud

I can please the Lord in every area of my life. He has begun a good work in me and will continue it. I choose to do all things without arguing or complaining. I am a child of God. I am important to the Lord and I am important in this world.

twelve

You're on the Right Track Now

Connie was afraid she would not be able to stay on the right track. She could never remember a time in her life when she didn't overeat. "I've never been thin," she said. "I think I was born fat. I've stayed fat my whole life. Saturdays and Sundays are the worst days for me. I usually stay in my room and eat and eat. I have cookies, chips and candy stashed in drawers, under my bed, in my closet—everywhere. Now that I've decided to slim down, I realize how bad my habits are."

Connie knew it would be hard, but she also knew the Lord was there helping her. "I must always remember that the Lord can change anything and anyone," Connie told us. "I believe that the Lord can show me how to be happy even if I seem like a hopeless case."

One Saturday afternoon when she was home alone, Connie went to the kitchen to find something to eat. But then she remembered Romans 12:2, "*Be a new and different person with a fresh newness in all you do and think.*" "I ate a small lunch of just a bowl of soup and one piece of toast. For me, that was really small because I have often eaten three or four sandwiches at one sitting."

"After I finished my *small* lunch, I was sitting there wondering what to do next. Suddenly I thought, '*Now open your book and do your Daily Power Time.*' "

Connie was delighted with herself that day because she felt

the Lord was speaking directly to her, and she could tell He was changing her habits and her desires. She didn't even reach for the cookies she knew were in the cookie jar. There was ice cream in the freezer but she didn't go near it. She read her lesson in *Slimming Down and Growing Up* and felt happier than she had felt in a long time.

Listening to the Lord

The Bible tells of Samuel, a boy who had dedicated his life to God. He wanted to follow God's ways and learn about Him. One night he was awakened by a voice calling his name. When he understood God was calling him, he answered immediately, "Speak, Lord, your servant is listening!"

Does the thought of God speaking to you sound strange? Sometimes people have the idea that God speaks only to special privileged ones, but that isn't true.

Neva Coyle, the founder of Overeaters Victorious and the *Free To Be Thin* program, was interviewed by a reporter from the *Chicago Daily News*. She told the reporter, "I ask the Lord what I'm supposed to eat and He tells me."

The reporter looked surprised. "Are you going to tell me that God *speaks* to you?"

Neva answered his question with another: "Are you going to tell me that water goes over Niagara Falls?"

"I don't see what that has to do with my question," the reporter said. "Water going over a falls is a natural event. It's a course of nature."

Smiling, Neva told him, "It's a natural event for God to speak to us, too."

"But surely He doesn't speak to just anybody!"

"But He does. God speaks to everybody. It's just that many people don't listen."

You hear God from deep within your own heart and your own thoughts. You don't have to be an adult to hear from God. You can be any age at all, any height at all, any weight at all.

You're on the right track when you're obeying the Lord through the power of His Holy Spirit. The Lord knows exactly what weight is best for *you*. Are you asking the Lord to help you reach the goal weight the chart on page 175 says is right for you?

You're on the right track, and you're doing great. Remember, the Lord himself is leading you. Psalm 103:14 (New International Version) says, *"He knows how we are formed."* That means He cares about your body and knows exactly how to help you be healthy and thinner. Will you trust Him?

Daily Power Time

Scripture Verse for Today:

"Your words are a flashlight to light the path ahead of me, and keep me from stumbling" (Psalm 119:105).

My thoughts today: ____________________

____

____

____

My special talk with God: ____________________

____

____

____

What today's Scripture verse means to me: ____________________

____

____

____

To Say Out Loud

God knows every bone in my body. He cares so much about me! I can follow His directions, like Samuel. I can obey His words and know that He is guiding me because He tells me so!

Just for Parents

You can help your child today by making overeating difficult to do. Don't have unhealthy foods in the cupboards or refrigerator where they are visible and easily accessible. Take an inventory of your cupboards and notice those foods you have stored which are clearly unhealthy. Your child probably thinks those nonnutritious foods are perfectly acceptable. One mother took a good look in her cupboards and was shocked to discover nearly everything there was loaded with preservatives, additives, artificial flavorings, and calories. She decided to help her child, and the rest of the family as well, by buying healthy foods.

Cooking and preparing meals that are low calorie and nutritious can be an exciting and creative experience. Making food attractive can be fun and rewarding. Unless your child loves to peel oranges, you might try cutting fruit into tasty bite-sized pieces rather than just handing your child a whole unpeeled orange for a snack. Or arrange fruit pieces in a small bowl with a dollop of yogurt on top.

Notice how you prepare food for your child. Minimize increasing calories in food by avoiding extra fats, coatings, or high-calorie sauces. Avoid frying in oil. If you fry or scramble eggs, use a non-stick pan. Your whole family will benefit by broiling, boiling and roasting your food, rather than frying or sautéing it. Research on weight control has shown that omitting just a single pat of butter or margarine daily can prevent the gain of three-and-one-half pounds in the course of a year! If you bread your meat, remember that a serving of bread must be removed from the rest of the day's calorie count.

Please know that we are praying for you. You have a big responsibility. We consider you a valuable person, and we want you to know you are not alone in your efforts to combat overweight. We care about you and will go on caring.

thirteen

Beware of the Sweets Trap

In your great-grandparents' day, food was often scarce in some parts of the world. Being thin might mean you were starving, and sick and poor. Parents longed to see their children with chubby, rosy cheeks, because that extra fat meant the children were getting plenty to eat. Fat meant healthy.

Carey's mother didn't live in a starving country, but just to be on the safe side, she made sure Carey ate enough to never be thin! By seventh grade, Carey was fatter than all his friends, but his parents weren't worried. At least he was healthy!

Then came the day the school sponsored a jog-a-thon, and everyone in Carey's class was required to take part. Carey thought he had practiced enough so on race day, he laced his tennis shoes and took off with the other forty-seven boys and girls along the short course. As they ran, Carey found out he wasn't so healthy after all. One by one the others flew by him as he struggled to lope along. It wasn't long before his whole body throbbed, and his breath became more pinched and painful. He gasped and wheezed and finally hobbled behind the others reaching the finish line long after the others. Then he stopped to go no further, while the rest of the joggers ran the course again and again. His fat, and all the sweets he ate to gain it, left him weak, not healthy.

You are learning the right way to become healthy—the way that works! Stuffing yourself with sweets isn't part of the best way to health. The Lord will not tell you to eat fattening sweets for energy, because the energy they give doesn't last. Jesus will not guide you to the candy store to pig out on chocolate. He knows that sweets are a trap, because you can get hooked on them. Anything too sweet, like candy bars, will never really quiet your hunger. All that sugar only makes you want to eat more of it.

God is teaching you how to take care of your body. Here are some tips to help you stay away from the sweets trap:

- If you must have something sweet, try having an orange before something sugary. You could even eat two oranges. Oranges have natural sugar and make you feel full far better than the sugary thing you crave.
- Drink water. Stop by your drinking fountain at school often during the day. After school when you are on your way home, and you're feeling an urge to snack, have a glass of water first.
- If you have a craving for something sweet, decide now how much of it you can afford to eat *before* you eat it. Remember your calorie limit for the day.
- Cookies, if they are not loaded with too much sugar, can be eaten. An oatmeal cookie (made with whole wheat flour) and fruit can be a tasty snack.
- Don't eat in secret. If you must have something sweet, eat it out in the open. Tell yourself, "I am in control," and write it down on your "What I Ate Today" sheet immediately.
- The sweet trap is only a trap if you let it be. If you allow yourself something sweet, tell yourself, "I will not overdo it. I will not eat until I'm stuffed. One scoop of ice cream tastes the same as three scoops."
- Tell yourself when you finished with your SMALL portion, "That's all I'm going to have. I'm done now."

If Jesus were here today, do you think He'd come home to His room, close the door behind Him, and then gorge on M & M's all by himself? Can you imagine Jesus going to the supermarket later for twelve banana cream pies, one for each disciple? Of course not!

You can be strong and stay clear of the sweets trap. You can *take charge*. As you do, you'll be on your way to the thin, healthy body you've always wanted.

Daily Power Time

The Lord gives us wisdom about how we are to eat. He is helping you now decide whether or not to eat sweets and unhealthy food. The Bible says, "*If you want to know what God wants you to do, ask him, and he will gladly tell you, for he is always ready to give a bountiful supply of wisdom to all who ask him. . .*" (James 1:5).

Scripture Verse for Today:

"*I will instruct you and teach you in the way you should go; I will counsel you and watch over you*" (Psalm 32:8).

My thoughts today: ____________________

____

____

____

My special talk with God: ____________________

____

____

____

What today's Scripture verse means to me: ____________________

____

____

____

To Say Out Loud

I can be happy eating smaller portions. I will beware of the sweets trap. The Lord is making me wise and watching over me.

fourteen

Taking Charge

After practice one day, the soccer team headed for a Mexican restaurant. While the other boys ordered heavy, fried, greasy foods, Tim chose a tostada salad without sour cream or guacamole. When the salad arrived, he ate the chicken, cheese, and lettuce, but not the fried shell it was served in.

His coach noticed, and told him later, "Hey, Tim, you're O.K. You're doing just great. I'm proud of you."

Tim was proud of himself, too. Not long ago he would have eaten the most fattening thing on the menu. When he had finished it, he would have cleaned up everyone else's leftovers, too.

Tim explained his new eating habits this way: "I never used to be in charge of what I ate. I just ate . . . and ate and ate and ate. Now I take charge."

Jamie Sticks to Her Decision

"Oh, come on, Jamie," her friend said temptingly, "just *one* piece of pizza won't hurt you." Jamie looked her straight in the eye and smiled. "No thanks," Jamie told her firmly. "Not today."

Jamie knew pizza wasn't on the daily plan she had made that morning, and didn't let her friend's urging lead her away from her plan. Jamie took charge and ordered a salad with lots of vegetables.

"Jamie," her friend said admiringly, "you really are serious about getting thin, aren't you? I wondered if you were going to stick with it, but now I see you really are!"

"And I'm going to make it," Jamie thought. Then she whispered a silent thanks to the Lord.

Carey and Terry Make Some Changes

Many overweight people overload on any food that's handy when they're hungry, whether it's good for them or not.

Carey said, "I found out I could get just as full eating fruit as I could stuffing myself on corn chips. In fact, corn chips never really filled me up. I used to eat them and *then* start eating other things."

"I remember eating bowl after bowl of cereal while watching a TV program," Terry said. "I'd eat big bowls of granola with bananas on top until I was stuffed. But by the time the next program came on, I was back at the refrigerator looking for something else to eat."

Jamie, Tim, Carey and Terry made up their minds to take charge of their eating habits. Terry doesn't stuff herself on bowls of cereal. Carey doesn't try to fill up on corn chips. Tim plans his meals. Jamie has learned to say no.

Your Powerhouse of Strength

You have a powerhouse of strength inside from the Holy Spirit who lives in you. When you become a Christian, the Holy Spirit of God takes up residence in your spirit and He gives you courage and strength. "*You, however, are controlled not by the sinful nature but by the Spirit, if the Spirit of God lives in you*" (Romans 8:9, NIV).

It's so wonderful to think about God's Spirit inside you. He is constantly urging, guiding, strengthening, teaching, and helping you. "*The spirit of him who raised Jesus from the dead is living in you. . .*" (Romans 8:11, NIV).

You can develop new strength because God's strength is within you. Your decision to grow thin may have been a hard one to make and it may seem like a hard one to keep. But when those moments of doubt come and you don't feel strong, remember the powerhouse within you. Turn to the Lord and tell Him your feelings right at that moment.

Taking Charge of Your Feelings

Unhappy feelings come to everyone sometimes. When you feel bad you might overeat to try to feel better. Then you feel even worse. You may even feel guilty. When Sara had bad feelings, she overate. But after she stuffed herself, she had another feeling to add to her anger—*guilt*.

Sara said the guilt made her feel hopeless about ever improving. "I'll never change. I'll always be fat," she would cry helplessly. Feeling guilty just made her want to eat more.

It's important to recognize your feelings. When you feel down, say to yourself: "*I feel sad but I won't overeat. I feel bad but I won't eat foods that aren't good for me.*"

You can be honest with Jesus when you feel like you can't stay on the right track. Jesus knows how to handle difficult matters. Tell the Lord your feelings. You may want to pray something like this, "Lord, I know I made a commitment to you, but I just don't care about staying on the right track now . . . I feel hurt (or angry or lonely), and I just want to eat something to make myself feel better."

The Lord understands. Your powerhouse is there ready for your use. The Lord is telling you: "The food will not comfort you. It will only make you feel worse. Listen to the truth. The truth is, you can be in charge. God is your comforter, not food."

The Word of God tells you, "*You will know the truth, and the truth will set you free*" (John 8:32).

While Jill was babysitting one evening, she decided she was hungry. She had already eaten three meals and two snacks for the day so she had one more snack to go. Her favorite ice cream was in the freezer. "Don't eat that ice cream," she heard coming from her heart. It was a thought she had, but she knew the Holy Spirit was speaking to her through her thought. She smiled. "Thank you, Lord," she said, taking an apple from the basket on the table to eat while doing her homework.

Will you pray this prayer now?

Lord, I'm on the right track now and I want to stay there. Hold me close to you. You are my powerhouse of strength. I know you love me and that's why I want to please you. I want to be good to my body for your sake. In Jesus' name, Amen.

Questions to Answer

1. My feelings are important. I will take the time to listen to my feelings. When I want to eat when I am not hungry, I will: ______________________________

2. When I want to eat chips or ice cream to stuff myself, I will remember: ______________________________

3. When I want to eat for comfort, I will remember my real Comforter is ______________________________.

True or False:

_____ When I am offered food that I have not planned to eat, it is O.K. for me to say no.
_____ Fat is something a person just "grows out of."
_____ If people make fun of me for changing my eating habits and getting thinner, I should just give up and quit.
_____ One of the traits of overweight people is to skip breakfast.
_____ One of the ways to get thin is to stop eating in secret.

Complete:

1. Some of my feelings after I stuff myself with food are:

____

2. Some of my feelings after I control what I eat are: _____

____

3. I feel good about myself when ______________________________. I feel guilty when ______________________________.

4. "*You will know the* _________, *and the* _________ *will set you free*" (John 8:32).

Daily Power Time

The Holy Spirit is your powerhouse. How can you be sure? The following verse tells you.

"You, however, are __________ not by the __________ nature but by the __________, if the __________ of God lives in you. . ." (Romans 8:9, NIV).

Scripture Verse for Today:

"For God has not given us a spirit of fear, but of power, and of love, and of a sound mind" (1 Timothy 1:7, NIV).

My thoughts today: ____________________

____

____

____

My special talk with God: ____________________

____

____

____

What today's Scripture verse means to me: __________

____

____

____

To Say Out Loud

- **I am a person who eats three meals a day.**
- **I am a person who eats two or three snacks a day.**
- **I am a person in charge of what I eat.**
- **I am a person who has power, love and self-discipline!**
- **I am on the right track!**

Just for Parents

Do you recognize your child's feelings? Can you tell if he is feeling sad, lonely, hurt, worried or misunderstood? Do you understand those angry outbursts your child engages in? Anger nearly always represents fear. Children are unable to recognize and handle negative emotions as easily as some adults, so your child may need your support to understand his feelings.

A child always patterns behavior after the behavior of his role models. How do you express anger? How do you express fear? If you are a screamer, you will likely have a child who is a screamer. If you have a temper, your child may display his feelings the same way. If you've had a problem with overweight and have dieted excessively without success, your child has seen the negative side of weight control.

God is there to help. We've talked about the Holy Spirit as a powerhouse within your child. That same Spirit is available to you, too.

Tips to Help Your Child

You and your child can both profit from talking about his "What I Ate Today" sheet. Going over it at the end of the day and then planning tomorrow's diet can help you both see patterns and needs. You might suggest new snacks and treats if this seems to be a problem area. Or increase your child's food awareness by inviting him to help shop for and prepare healthy foods. However, don't take your child food shopping if he is hungry. Eat something nutritious first and then go shopping.

Help your child to avoid temptation without being obvious. Don't visit friends and family without telling them in advance of your child's needs. It's not fair to bring him to Grandma's if she will overwhelm him with offers of sweets, and then be hurt if he doesn't gorge himself as he has in the past.

It would be almost cruel to take your child to a ballgame and then warn him he'd better not eat peanuts when everyone else is eating them. PLAN AHEAD. Try, "Honey, we're going to the ballgame tomorrow. Should we bring snacks from home so we don't have to eat the stuff they serve at the ballpark?"

If your child says he'd really rather have a hot dog and peanuts, then add these to tomorrow's food plan. If your child plans for them, he can enjoy eating without guilt.

Remember, it is not YOU who is in control of your child's behavior. Your child is learning to control his *own* behavior. You could tape your child's mouth shut and he would lose weight, but weight loss is not our only goal. More important are self-control and confidence in God. We believe your child has the ability to succeed in his own strength with the Lord. Of course, your help and encouragement will make that success come easier, but your "encouragement" does not mean you must become a police officer. You must not police your child's eating habits, or nag him.

Consider yourself blessed to have a child who cares enough to work toward getting thin. Your child is blessed, too, to have your support. Our prayer is that the Lord will draw you and your child closer through the loving guidance of the Holy Spirit as you work toward your common goal. We know, as thousands of adults on the *Free To Be Thin* program have attested, that when you reach "Maintenance" with your child, you will say, "We've gotten much more than *thin* out of this venture." (Read our book, *There's More to Being Thin Than Being Thin* for additional insights.)

May God touch you both with sweetness and compassion today.

fifteen

What Makes You Hungry?

Have you ever heard of "hunger pangs"? They are contractions of the stomach telling you when you're hungry. It takes just a few bites of food (like just a *third* of a banana) to stop real hunger pangs.

But there's another feeling that often gets mixed up with real hunger; we call it your "appetite hunger," or craving. A craving is the feeling that pushes you to eat whether your body really needs more food or not. Maybe Jill didn't feel hungry before she walked into the restaurant where her mother worked, but when she smelled those aromas coming from the kitchen, she said, "My mouth just watered, and I could taste everything, just by the smell." She felt like she *had* to have something to eat. It's that unnecessary eating that caused Jill to become as fat as she was.

Your body asks for only enough food to be healthy and strong. What you crave is usually all the extras, the things you don't need. When you crave something to eat, just a little bit of it won't do. You may start with one bite, but then not stop until you've finished every crumb, whether you are hungry or not. Even if she wasn't hungry, Jill could still eat a whole meal, complete with milk and bread. Her craving was triggered by a hunger that wasn't real.

Different people get cravings from different things. Terry said the smell of breakfast cooking made her drool, but Bonnie told us, "The one thing I can't stand is the smell of food in the morning. Ugh! It makes me sick!" Bonnie's friend, Betsy, said, "I really can't stand the smells coming from the kitchen in the restaurant. For some reason it reminds me of when I had chicken pox. I hate it." If a smell can make one person feel hungry, and another feel sick, that means cravings aren't real hunger, and you can control and change them.

Do certain smells, like popcorn popping, make you begin to crave food even if you aren't hungry? What kinds of food do you especially crave? If you know, you can learn to control your cravings. You won't get rid of them completely, but you can learn to take charge of them.

Tim and the Candy-Bar Victory

Tim wanted a candy bar after school in the worst way. He was practically drooling when he got to the counter at the corner market. His eyes were locked on the chocolate bars on the shelf in front of him. His feelings said, "Candy!" His mind said, "Why not?" But his spirit said, "No way!" Tim had not planned on candy that day. His snacks included quesadillas and frozen yogurt, so he told himself, "No way," and left the candy bars alone.

Tim won the battle with his craving that day. He decided he'd have a candy bar tomorrow as one of his snacks after he fit it in his daily food plan.

The next morning as he made his food plan, he figured out that the candy bar had 380 calories. He could budget that into his daily allowance by cutting out dessert at dinner and having two apples for his other snack. He would not eat butter or fried foods, and he would have his salad without cheese on top. Now he was in control. When Tim ate a candy bar that afternoon he did not have to eat it in secret, or feel guilty.

You can control your cravings like Tim did. Here are some tips to help:

- Don't deny yourself the foods you enjoy. *Control them instead.*
- Your appetite is different from anyone elses. Get to know

the foods you like best. Write them down.

- If you crave something fattening, work it into your daily plan. Go ahead and have it, but write it on your "What I Ate Today" sheet immediately.
- When you feel like having something to eat, but you really aren't hungry and what you want isn't on your daily plan, STOP!
- Tell yourself you'll have that certain something tomorrow. It's not on your plan for today so you aren't having it. Tell yourself no.

Only Bread for Dinner?

Carey's special craving was bread, and he ate lots of it, but all that bread was only adding to Carey's weight problem. However, Carey really liked bread, so we told him not to do away with it completely, and he didn't. With our O.K., sometimes for dinner Carey would eat nothing but bread and a glass of milk.

Maybe that doesn't sound healthy, and if Carey ate only bread for a long period, it wouldn't be. But Carey was learning to listen to his own special food desires and make room for them. He *planned* to eat the bread and only ate as many slices as his calorie limit would allow. He helped make sure he didn't go over his calorie limit for the day by cutting out toast at breakfast, and skipping the potato salad he would have had for lunch. Instead of denying his craving, or giving in to his craving, he learned to take charge of it.

Instead of your appetite being an enemy, pushing you to stuff yourself, you can change your appetite into a friend by taking charge of it. Here's how:

1. *Listen to your appetite.* What are you craving and when?

2. *Plan for your appetite.* Don't ignore your cravings or try to deny them. Your appetite is not a horrible monster out to get you. It's something you can live with and control.

3. *Let your appetite have its way WITH CONTROL.* When you know you want a certain food at a certain time of day, schedule it as one of your three snacks, or make an entire meal of it. BUT COUNT THE CALORIES AND DON'T EXCEED

YOUR CALORIE ALLOWANCE FOR THE DAY.

4. *Ask God to make your appetite what He wants it to be.* If God is in charge of your life, He wants to be in charge of all of it. He wants to be Lord of your appetite as well as Lord of your thoughts and goals. He wants to be good to every part of you—even your appetite.

Remember that you're in control now. In the past you may not have been able to control your eating urges, but now you can. You may eat without guilt because you control how much and when you eat. You don't have to give up jelly beans for the rest of your life. The only thing you're giving up is lack of control.

Will you pray this prayer?

> Dear Lord, I give you my appetite. I will not be ashamed and I will not feel guilty for the foods I crave. I will dedicate my appetite to you and trust you to remind me of my promise to eat with a plan and with control. Thank you for my powerhouse, the Holy Spirit, to help me. In Jesus' name, Amen.

Questions to Answer

Check one:

1. My appetite is something I can: _____ control; _____ not do a thing about.

2. My appetite depends upon: _____ what I tell myself about food; _____ how hungry I am.

3. I have a "good" appetite because: _____ I don't overeat; _____ I overeat.

Answer:

1. Many overweight people can't tell when they are hungry. Can you describe your feelings when you're hungry? ________

____

2. Describe the difference between "hunger pangs" and "cravings": ______________________________________

3. When you want to eat something you really like, even though it's fattening, you can include it in your diet. How do you do this?

4. What are the four ways you can make your appetite your friend?

a.

b.

c.

d.

5. Have you asked God to control your appetite today?

Daily Power Time

Scripture Verse for Today:

(Jesus said) "*If anyone loves me, he will obey my teachings. My Father will love him, and we will come to him and make our home with him*" (John 14:23, NIV).

My thoughts today:

My special talk with God:

What today's Scripture verse means to me: ____________

To Say Out Loud

I can control my appetite. God cares about all of me. He cares about my appetite. He loves me and lives in me.

sixteen

Changing Your Mind About Food

When your favorite football or basketball team goes out to play a game, the team wants just one thing: they want to win! Everyone around them joins forces to help. The coach talks to the team about winning. The cheerleaders sing and cheer and yell about winning. The crowds in the stands wave banners and shout to encourage the team to win.

Now imagine this. Your favorite team still wants to win. But before the game, their coach says, "You've lost games before, so you can plan on losing this one, too." The cheerleaders' first yell is "L-O-S-E! We're gonna lose, lose, lose!" And the people in the stands ask each other, "How many points do you think they'll lose by today?"

With all those people helping them think about losing, do you think it would be easier or harder for the team members to play their best? Harder, of course!

As you fight against fat, your thoughts about food are like a cheerleader in your mind. What cheer do you choose your cheerleader will yell? Do you say, "Good for you. You're gonna win over fat!" Or do you say, "Poor you. Everybody else is loading up on the gooey cake. You only get this plain old apple. They get all the good stuff." A cheerleader like that certainly won't make eating God's way easier.

Change your mind about food. You can tell yourself the truth. You want to be thin and strong, right? Then it's important to tell yourself that greasy and fattening foods are *not* delicious or wonderful, and that sweet gooey foods are *not* terrific.

Some people call rich and fattening foods "yummie" and "out of this world." One food that is bad for you and loaded with sugar and chemicals calls itself "heavenly." There's nothing heavenly about it! Heavenly food is healthy and is good for your body. Heavenly food is not loaded with sugar and chemicals that leave you fatter and weaker.

Now that you're growing up and slimming down, you don't have to just "endure" through eating the right food. Tell yourself salads are crisp and crunchy and terrific. Tell yourself broiled chicken is wonderful. Stop wishing you were having a malted milk instead of the glass of orange juice you chose. You tell yourself that you'd rather have the clean, healthy feeling orange juice gives you, instead of loading your body with all the gloppy fat and sugar in a malted milk you hadn't planned on.

The *Slimming Down and Growing Up* program is not something to do just until you get thin, and then forget about. You want to be good to your body for the rest of your life. Later in this book, you'll read the Bible story of Daniel, a young person who chose to eat God's way. You'll discover that Daniel didn't eat his special diet just for ten days, and then on the day he reached his goal, gobble up all the food he hadn't been eating. His eating plan lasted for life.

Your new way of eating will last for life, too, because you're not dieting; you're learning to eat God's way. God doesn't intend you will live the rest of your life eating only lettuce leaves. You'll still have malted milks once in a while, but now you are in control of how much you have, and when you have them. You are now free to say, "That's enough."

You're free to make happy, healthy choices. Tell yourself, "A crisp, juicy apple tastes great, and it's good for your body, too."

Adults can make mistakes in how they think about food. One mother may say, "My son has a *good* appetite because he eats so much." Another mother says, "My son eats so little. He has such a *bad* appetite." They're saying their sons are good if they eat a lot.

But what if the son who has such a "good" appetite is overweight! Is his appetite really so good? Maybe his mother should change the expression around to say, "My son has a *bad* appetite because he eats so much." Adults and kids both need to learn a new way of thinking about food, and about other things, too.

Terry Thinks a New Way About Moving—and Loses Weight!

Terry's home in Ohio always buzzed with people and fun. When she came home from school, her grandma, or her aunt and baby cousins would be in the kitchen, visiting her mother. Weekends meant happy times with relatives. It seemed like there was always someone to talk to or play with, and no time to be bored.

Then Terry's dad announced his company was giving him a different job in California. He tried to make it sound great, with the ocean, and the fruit trees, and being able to barbecue outside all winter long. But Terry's mother cried, and Terry felt like moving had to be the worst thing that could ever happen to her.

"After we moved my mother started working, and I came home from school to an empty house," Terry said. "It made me sad, so I'd head for the kitchen, put my books down on the counter, and start eating. Then I'd go to bed. I didn't want to do anything but eat and sleep.

"Saturdays in our new home were lonely and scary. All I wanted to do was eat, watch cartoons on TV, and eat some more." Terry had always liked food and taken second helpings, but now she ate third and fourth helpings at meals, besides all the overeating between meals.

Even more than lonely, Terry felt angry. She was mad at God for letting her father get transferred. It just wasn't fair that such a terrible thing had happened to her. Terry wanted God to fit into *her* plan. She was angry because He didn't do what she wanted Him to. He wouldn't answer her prayers to have her father transferred back to Ohio. He wouldn't make everything like it was before.

Then one Sunday at Terry's new church, the pastor talked about a Bible verse Terry had never understood before.

"We know that all that happens to us is working for our good if we love God and are fitting into his plans" (Romans 8:28).

The pastor explained that bad things that happen to us can turn out to be *good*, not bad, if we trust God to make good from them. Terry listened carefully. Could it be that there might be good for her in this move to California? It all seemed so terrible, but maybe if she asked God's help, He could help her find the good things He had planned for her in it. She asked God to forgive her for being angry, and asked Him to help her like California.

Fitting into God's Plan

With her new attitude, Terry began to feel expectant instead of angry. She became friendlier at school. She began working harder at her studies, and was nicer to her parents. To fit into God's plan for her eating, she joined the *Free To Be Thin* group her mother attended. When the ladies asked if she minded being the only youngster in the group, Terry would say, "I don't mind. I'm getting thin God's way." And she did grow to be the thin, happy girl she wanted to be.

When Terry decided to change her angry thoughts, her feelings began to change. Once she decided to tell herself, "God will make all things work for good because He says so in His Word," her feelings began to change for the better. Now she's lost her anger and her extra weight, too!

Everybody feels sad sometimes. It's not terrible to feel sad. It's not terrible to feel angry either, or unhappy. All these feelings come as a part of life, and everyone feels them sometimes. But these bad feelings don't have to be permanent.

You can make them change by saying in your thoughts, "God is with me. He loves me and is helping me."

You can think new thoughts about food, and about the bad things that happen to you. As you do, you're fitting into God's plan for you. With right thoughts, you'll find that good, healthy foods can become "yummy" to you. Like Terry, you'll see God working good for you in situations you used to think had nothing good about them.

Questions to Answer

1. Terry, at the beginning of this chapter, overate when she felt lonely and sad. What do you think she should have done instead? ______________________________

____

True or False:

_____ Everyone feels sad sometimes.
_____ When you feel down the Lord is ready to help you.
_____ Bad feelings are not permanent.
_____ Overeating will help you feel better.

Daily Power Time

Scripture Verse for Today:

"*Remember, when someone wants to do wrong it is never God who is tempting him, for God never wants to do wrong and never tempts anyone else to do it*" (James 1:13).

My thoughts today: ______________________________

____

____

____

My special talk with God: ______________________________

____

____

____

What today's Scripture verse means to me: ______________________________

____

To Say Out Loud

Bad things that happen can be turned to good if I pray and ask God's forgiveness and help. God helps me understand my feelings and know myself better. He never tempts me to do wrong. He gives me a happy heart and not a sad one.

Just for Parents

Certain activities, like going to the movies, often trigger an eating response. You may not be hungry, but still you stop at the refreshment counter to load up with popcorn, candy and drinks before sitting down to watch the movie. Or you may be at a fair or circus. Even if you just finished lunch, you may stop and buy cotton candy, ice cream or some other treat to eat during the festivities. Thanksgiving means pumpkin pie; Halloween means candy; birthdays call for cake, hungry or not.

We are not saying to stop these eating practices. Eating and certain activities seem to go hand in hand. It would seem rare indeed to spend an afternoon at the zoo without stopping for a refreshment. What we have stressed is to recognize the difference between real hunger and cravings, and to make room for controlled cravings.

Will you recognize your own responses to appetite and hunger? Do you eat indiscriminately and without control? How much does real hunger have to do with the food you choose to eat?

Slimming Down and Growing Up teaches your child not to try to wipe out the part of his personality responsible for eating. Rather, he needs to understand himself and his eating behavior, and then learn new and better ways of eating and meeting needs. That's why we don't ask you to remove every trace of sugar or starch from your kitchen now that your child is learning new habits. He needs to know sugar will always be around in this world but that it is possible to live sensibly with it.

You can deal with food cravings, and with special-occasion eating by simply planning ahead. Be aware of the food being eaten. Your child is learning lifetime habits now, and it is imperative that he be aware of what he eats. If a licorice stick at the park and a taco at a party are not counted as bona-fide eating, all is defeated. Most overweight people eat unconsciously throughout the day. Children can be the worst offenders because they are not fully aware of their bodies.

Since many of our cravings are triggered by the smells of

food, you can begin to retrain your sense of smell. Play a game with your child where each of you sees how many "favorite smells" you can come up with and *none* can be food. After identifying the smells, discuss what these smells make you think of, or how they make you feel. One child whose father was a construction worker said, "I like the smell of Daddy when he comes home from work. It makes me think of huge machines and big things, and then my daddy is as big as they are."

Yesterday's Scripture verse, John 14:23, reminds us of the precious relationship we have with God. How fortunate you are to have the love of God filling you and flooding your home. Our prayer is that *Slimming Down and Growing Up* is enhancing the love relationship between all the members of your family.

seventeen

Do You Have to Be Big to Be Strong?

To Carey, his dad always seemed as big as a giant. When Carey was a little boy, his mother encouraged him to eat so he would grow up big and strong like his dad, and that sounded great to Carey! So Carey tried to eat as much as his dad so he'd be sure to get as big.

At thirteen, Carey was shorter than most kids his age, and all that food couldn't make him grow any taller. It only made him get wider. Overeating hadn't made him strong and tough like he hoped it would, either. With that extra fat, he couldn't run fast, or lift heavy things, or keep up with the other kids.

Carey began his *Slimming Down and Growing Up* eating plan, and started growing thin. But as he did, he began to worry. He was already short. If he got thinner, would he be a weakling? Would he look like a sissy?

Carey had to learn that thin people can be very strong. It's not necessary to be big to be strong. You don't even have to wait until you're an adult to be strong.

The Bible tells us in 1 Samuel 17 about two big, tall men who turned out to be weak, and a young, thin boy named David who proved he could be stronger than both of them.

David, the Teen-age Hero

When David was a teen-ager, the king of his country, Saul, led the army of Israel to war against the Philistines. Seven of

David's older brothers were soldiers in Saul's army, so one day David's father told him to take them some food.

When David arrived at the outskirts of the army camp, King Saul's soldiers were just heading for the battlefield to take on the Philistines. As the two armies stood facing each other, a Philistine giant named Goliath stepped out and challenged any of Saul's men to come and fight him. But the soldiers of Israel took one look at the size of that giant and ran in terror back to their camp.

Goliath was big—over nine feet tall. That's probably taller than the ceiling in your house. He was as powerful as he was tall. On his shoulders and chest he wore huge, heavy armor. He wore bronze leggings and a bronze helmet, and flashed an enormous sword. All this armor weighed almost two hundred pounds, yet Goliath wore it like it weighed nothing. King Saul was big, too (nearly *seven* feet tall), and one of the biggest men in all of Israel.

David was not big. He was not even a soldier, like his brothers. He was a simple boy who watched sheep and played music on his harp. But David understood that real strength doesn't depend on your size; it depends on your trust in God.

When he saw King Saul and the Israeli army running away from Goliath, he asked, "Who is this heathen Philistine, anyway, that he is allowed to defy the armies of the living God?" Pretty brave talk for a young shepherd boy, don't you think? David's oldest brother didn't think so. He just thought David was showing off and acting like a brat. "What are you doing around here," he asked David angrily. "What about the sheep you're supposed to be taking care of?"

But instead of arguing with his brother, or pouting and going back to his sheep, David went to the king. "Don't you worry about a thing," he told Saul confidently. "*I'll* take care of this Philistine!"

King Saul must have thought poor little David was crazy. The king told him not to be ridiculous. "How can a boy like you fight with a giant? You're only a boy and he has been in the army *since* he was a boy!"

But David wouldn't change his mind, so the king consented to let him try to fight Goliath.

When David faced the giant, he had no armor, and he carried no spear or shield. Goliath was furious that Israel would insult him by sending this young boy to fight him. He cursed David and shouted that he would give David's flesh to the birds and wild animals to eat.

But David took his little shepherd's sling and rushed at the giant with this shout, "You come to me with a sword and spear, but I come to you in the name of the Lord of the armies of heaven and of Israel!" He shouted, "Today the Lord will conquer you. I will kill you and cut off your head. He will give you to us!"

With that, David let fly a stone from his slingshot, and struck the giant right between the eyes. Goliath fell to the ground, dead.

Being nine feet tall couldn't save Goliath when he faced David's faith in God. King Saul's size didn't make him strong, either. It was David's giant-size trust in God, not his size, that made him the strongest of all.

Can you see yourself as David saw himself? Instead of worrying about his small size, David fearlessly declared to Goliath, "*I come to you in the name of the Lord.*" If you love and trust the Lord, you can feel strong, just as David did, no matter what size you are.

Questions to Answer

1. When you read how David conquered Goliath, where does true strength come from? ______________________

2. Do you think all Christians can be like David? ________ Why? ______________________________

Daily Power Time

Scripture Verse for Today:

"*Anything is possible if you have faith*" (Mark 9:23).

My thoughts today: ______________________________

____

____

My special talk with God: ____________________

____

____

____

What today's Scripture verse means to me: ____________________

____

____

____

To Say Out Loud

I will not call myself weak or fat again. I will see myself with God's eyes. Because the Lord is strong I can be strong. Like David, I am strong in the name of the Lord.

eighteen

Overeating and Special People

Jamie wasn't the only overweight person in her family. Her father, her mother, and both her brothers all ate too much and weighed too much. Her mother's doctor had even told Jamie's mother that she must lose weight for her health's sake. Slimming down and growing up in an overweight family created three special problems for Jamie.

First, it was hard to be different from the rest of the family. Eating had been one of her family's main things to enjoy together. Mealtimes were important, and everyone looked forward to her mother's good cooking. One of the family's ways to say "I love you" to their mother had been to eat two, three, or four helpings of the delicious food she fixed. Jamie felt a part of the family's special times when she ate almost as much as her older brothers. Now, when Jamie said no to the big slices of pie piled high with ice cream everyone else was eating, she felt different.

Also, it was hard to be growing thin without making the others feel she thought she was better than they. She wondered if they thought she felt she was *right* for getting thin, and they were wrong. She did worry about her mother's health, too. Should she tell her mother it was wrong to eat so many rich foods? Jamie wasn't sure.

Another difficult time was when her brothers would tease her and make fun of her for not eating as much as she did before.

Jamie tackled her problems the right way. She began by writing a prayer to God during her Daily Power Time. She wrote:

"Dear Lord, help me to be an example to my family. Help me to show them how much I love them, and how much you love them. They tease me for not eating so much anymore, and Mom's feelings were hurt last night because I didn't have any pie. I don't want my family mad at me. Please help them to understand, and help me to be a good daughter and sister. Love, Jamie."

After she prayed, Jamie decided to try explaining her feelings to her family. One night at the dinner table she said, "I'm serious about getting thin. I'm really going to be working hard to change my eating habits. It's not going to be easy. Mom is such a good cook and I like to eat. But I'm going to work at cutting down. I just want you all to know."

She didn't tell them they ought to lose weight, too, or that she was the only one in the family who was right about food, and all the rest were wrong. She didn't make her mother feel bad by saying all that rich food she served was making them unhealthy. She let her family know that the problem was *hers*, and *she* was going to change, and asked their help.

When her brothers teased her (one told her she'd never make it), she didn't throw a fit, but she didn't quit eating right, either. Instead, Jamie trusted the Lord and continued to expect His help, even if her brothers didn't help her.

Jamie had to deal with her Aunt Martha, too, during a visit to her home. Aunt Martha had just baked some éclairs and offered one to Jamie, but Jamie refused. "I'm becoming a new me," Jamie explained. "Don't you want to see me thinner?"

"Just one little éclair won't hurt you, will it?" her aunt coaxed.

"Aunt Martha," Jamie said in a firm voice, "maybe after I become thinner I'll be able to eat one of your éclairs. Right now I can't because it's not on my food plan today. But I would love to have an apple if you have one."

When her aunt saw Jamie's determination, she began to cooperate. Instead of rich pastries, she had fresh fruit salads and light treats ready when Jamie visited. Being kind, but honest, with her aunt paid off for Jamie.

If your family is overweight, here are some ideas to help you know what to say (and not say) to them:

1. Explain in a loving way that you have decided to change your eating habits to become thinner and healthier for the Lord.
2. Remember, becoming thin does not make a person better than someone else who chooses to stay fat.
3. Thin people are *not* right and fat people are *not* wrong.
4. Becoming thin is a decision *you* have made. It's yours alone. You're not overeating anymore, but you can't force others not to overeat. Don't try to change anyone but yourself.
5. Pray and ask the Lord to make you a loving example to those you care about.

Daily Power Time

Scripture Verse for Today:

"*And let us not get tired of doing what is right, for after a while we will reap a harvest of blessing if we don't get discouraged and give up*" (Galatians 6:9).

My thoughts today: ____________________

____

____

____

My special talk with God: ____________________

____

____

____

What today's Scripture verse means to me: ____________________

____

To Say Out Loud

I can be loving and kind to others, even if they are eating the kinds of food I don't choose to eat. I can be a good example and not get discouraged.

Just for Parents

Your child is probably more tempted to overeat at home than any other place. A child's experiences with Mother cooking a feast in the kitchen, then all the family around the table with food as the main attraction form deeply implanted associations. But home should not mean food to us.

Each of the items listed are times of temptations to overeat. You can be more aware of your family's habits and your child's overeating problem if you recognize the patterns set in your home and the behavior you model to your child.

Check if you do any of the following:

_____ Eat while watching TV.
_____ Eat while driving the car.
_____ Eat while studying or doing paperwork.
_____ Eat while reading.
_____ Eat while on the job.
_____ Eat while shopping.
_____ Eat while preparing a meal.
_____ Eat when cleaning up after a meal.
_____ Eat more alone than with others.
_____ Eat before going to bed.
_____ Get out of bed in the middle of the night to eat.
_____ Eat more on weekends than during the week.
_____ Eat more in the evening than during the day.
_____ Skip breakfast but stuff yourself later on in the day.

This checklist was not designed to make you feel guilty, but to give you more understanding into the psychology of overeating. Your child will tend to eat as you eat. If you eat while watching TV, it will be hard for your child not to eat while watching TV.

You may need to change some habits. Perhaps your family needs to look together at how important food is in your home. Deciding on some activities and reactions that do not center around eating could be a positive change for your whole family.

nineteen

Talking to Yourself

Did you know you are sending messages to yourself all the time? Sometimes you talk out loud, but most of the time you talk silently to yourself. You may say something like, "So *there's* my blue notebook. I thought I lost it." Or you may be all alone and ask a question like, "I wonder what time it is?" or "Where did I put my toothbrush?"

Tim talked out loud to himself the morning he tried out for the soccer team at school. As he sat on the edge of his bed pulling his socks on, he said, "I hope I make it. I wonder if Joe Peabody will be there. I wonder if Melissa Gordon will be watching. What if I don't make it and Melissa laughs at me . . . Oh!"

Tim doesn't remember all the things he said to himself that day or most days. Most of us can't remember much of what we tell ourselves. Melissa Gordon didn't remember when she asked herself out loud, "Will Tim notice me at the tryouts? Will he realize that I came just to cheer for him?"

Talking to Yourself Silently

When you talk to yourself silently, you're *thinking*. There are many different kinds of thinking. There's happy thinking, sad thinking, worried thinking. Your thoughts can be learning thoughts, imagination thoughts, daydreaming thoughts, or praying thoughts. All of your thinking is important, because your thoughts can help you grow thin if you know what to tell yourself.

Imagining Is Talking to Yourself

Did you ever imagine you were somebody else or somewhere else? Did you ever dream you were a hero everybody admired and respected? This thinking is called *imagining*. It's fun to imagine you're somebody different or that you're the greatest hero around. It's fun to make up stories and pretend. It's fun to use our imaginations.

Imagining means "What if?" When you imagine you're successful, you're saying, "What if I succeed?" Then the more you think about it, the more you tell yourself, "Yes, I *will* succeed." Tell yourself, "I can imagine myself successful at getting thin because the Lord is with me. The Lord gives me confidence and strength."

Let's imagine now. Imagine that you're exactly the size you want to be. Imagine you're eating three meals a day and three snacks. Imagine yourself confident and content. Imagine not staying angry or hurt. Imagine running and playing sports. Imagine you're strong and healthy.

Now imagine yourself sitting at a table with all of your favorite foods. Imagine yourself taking small portions for your plate. Imagine yourself saying no to second helpings. Imagine yourself chewing slowly and taking sips of your water or milk as you eat. Imagine yourself feeling relaxed and not even wanting to stuff yourself.

Now imagine yourself looking in the cupboard for something to eat. On the shelf you see some cookies, cereal, crackers, bread and chips, but you close the cupboard door without taking anything out to eat. You tell yourself, "I won't eat anything from the cupboard."

Imagine yourself opening the refrigerator instead, and taking out a juicy ripe peach and a plump sweet plum. Imagine your mouth watering over a tasty bowl of fresh fruit with a luscious strawberry on top.

This kind of imagining is *planning for success*. Fill your thoughts with thoughts of doing well. Imagine yourself doing well, not only in your eating habits but in all things.

Many people imagine themselves failing. Have you ever

heard somebody say, "Oh, I'm just a dumb head. I couldn't do that." Or "Nobody likes me." Maybe you have said these things. Maybe you have told yourself negative things that aren't true. It's important to control your thoughts and the things you tell yourself. Planning to succeed and imagining yourself successful are ways to help you.

Imagine yourself in the kitchen when your mother is preparing dinner. Can you imagine not nibbling before dinner? When you nibble before or after dinner you are adding a lot of calories to your body. The extra nibbling you do through the day may all add up to another whole meal. Imagine yourself waiting to sit down at the table before nibbling. Imagine yourself after the meal, too. If there are leftovers, see yourself not eating them unless you have planned to eat them.

Just one lick of peanut butter from a spoon, cake crumbs from the cake pan, the last of the gravy in the pan, the teensy taste of leftover macaroni—all of this food adds up. It's important to have a picture of yourself in your mind not nibbling before and after meals.

Imagining is one way you talk to yourself and *learning* is another way. You become what you tell yourself over and over. Habits are learned. You learned to overeat, but now you are learning not to overeat. You are becoming healthier, thinner and smarter, too.

Questions to Answer

True or False:

_____ Nearly every minute of the day you are saying something to yourself.
_____ When you talk to yourself silently, you're thinking.
_____ Imagining success starts by asking "What if?"
_____ *Imagining* can be a good kind of talking to yourself.

Complete:

"I can imagine myself successful at getting thin because

____

____

____."

Daily Power Time

When you imagine yourself doing well, you will help yourself succeed. If you picture yourself not doing well, you help yourself fail. Your thoughts are important!

Scripture Verse for Today:

"*May my spoken words and unspoken thoughts be pleasing even to you, O Lord my Rock and my Redeemer*" (Psalm 19:14).

My thoughts today: ______________________________

____

____

____

My special talk with God: ___________________________

____

____

____

What today's Scripture verse means to me: ______________

____

____

____

To Say Out Loud

I picture myself a success on my *Slimming Down and Growing Up* program. I will tell myself good things, not unhappy, sad things. I will not allow evil or gloomy word pictures in my mind or thoughts.

twenty

A Wisdom Quiz

Young people tell us things like, "I used to be really stupid about eating." "I used to eat everything and anything without even thinking about what I put into my mouth." "I was not at all smart. Even my baby sister was smarter than me. She ate healthy baby food but I ate fattening junk foods that didn't make me feel good or healthy."

Being wise means able to reason and think properly about what is true or right. When you make a *wise decision,* it shows that you have the ability to choose what is true and right.

Being wise is something you *learn* how to be. How do you learn to be wise? God gives us wisdom. He gives us thoughts that are true and good. When you decided to eat new foods to help your body become strong and healthy, you began learning to be wise. You are learning God's way to eat.

Your goal is an important one, and the way to reach it is to use your wisdom.

Here is a sample daily diet. Read it and see if you can tell why one side is wise and the other not so wise.

Meal	Not So Wise	Wise
Breakfast	Frozen waffles; syrup; chocolate milk	Scrambled eggs; whole grain toast; orange juice

Snack	Package of chocolate cream-filled cupcakes	Whole fresh apple or other tasty fruit
Lunch	Big Mac; french fries; chocolate shake	Salad; tuna fish sandwich; (whole-grain bread); carrot sticks; frozen yogurt
Snack	Two popsicles	Oatmeal cookies; milk
Dinner	Frozen TV dinner; bread and butter	Roast chicken; steamed vegetables; baked potato; salad; fresh strawberries
Snack	Salted peanuts	Apple juice; Banana

Think about eating wisely. On the "Not so wise" side of the page you will notice a big difference from the "wise" side. Most of the "not so wise" food is unhealthy, sugary, starchy and too salty. Start out on your own adventure to find out about foods and why they are "wise" or "unwise."

Your Body Needs Vitamins

You gain energy and strength eating foods like fresh fruits and vegetables, chicken, fish, whole-grain breads, milk, cheeses and juices.

Your Body Needs Minerals

You become stronger and healthier when you don't eat lots of junk food and sweets. There are minerals in fruits, vegetables, meat, fish, poultry, dairy and wheat products.

You can learn to eat and enjoy foods with the vitamins and minerals your body needs.

Your Body Needs Protein

Protein is important in every meal. Protein gives you energy. Protein is found in fish, poultry, eggs, cheese, milk and yogurt. There is also protein in beans, seeds, nuts and whole-grain cereals.

Because you are still growing, your body especially needs protein. Many times when people try to lose weight, they cut out important foods. They miss out on protein, vitamins and minerals. They may lose weight, but they also lose good health.

Tell yourself, "I will not eat to hurt myself. I will eat to be healthy."

"*Let your eyes look straight ahead, fix your gaze directly before you*" (Proverbs 4:25, NIV).

You have made an important decision to succeed, and you will do it. You gain strength from the Word of God. Speak the Word of God out loud to yourself by repeating the Bible verse you just read. The Lord is telling you in His Word to look straight ahead at what is true. When your gaze is fixed straight in front of you, you are not allowing yourself to wallow here and there thinking about foods you know will hurt you. When you think of food, you think of healthy, happy, food that will make your body strong.

Questions to Answer

1. God gives us wisdom. Wisdom is: ____________________

____

2. Name some foods your body needs to stay healthy:

____

____

3. Psalm 119:1 says, "*Happy are all who perfectly follow the laws of God.*" The "law" of God means all of God's revealed will. God wants you to know His will for you concerning food and your eating habits. He wants you to delight in keeping your eating habits according to the Word.

"*How can a young . . . [person] stay pure? By reading your*

[God's] Word and following its rules" (Psalm 119:9).

How can you keep your way pure? ____________________

Daily Power Time

Scripture Verse for Today:

"*Bless me with life so that I can continue to obey you. Open my eyes to see wonderful things in your Word. I am but a pilgrim here on earth: how I need a map—and your commands are my chart and guide. I long for your instructions more than I can tell*" (Psalm 119:17–20).

My thoughts today: ____________________

____

____

____

____

My special talk with God: ____________________

____

____

____

____

What today's Scripture verse means to me: ____________________

____

____

____

____

To Say Out Loud

Thank you, Lord, for giving me a chart and guide. Thank you for instructing me. Thank you for making me wise and showing me how to understand myself and my thoughts. Thank you for showing me how to eat so that I can be strong and healthy.

Just for Parents

We want to share with you these words from Virginia and Norman Rohrer in their little book, *Junk Food.*[1] The Rohrers ask you to give your family a gift of love, and we couldn't agree more. Whether you are young or old, male or female, consider these resolutions and let them be your special legacy.

1. Establish early a reverence for food as a beautiful gift from a loving Creator.
2. Expose children to a great variety of wholesome food. Let them experience and enjoy all types of flavors and textures of food.
3. Let them see Mother and Dad relish natural food. Discourage criticism of wholesome food.
4. Don't give food as a reward or withhold it as punishment. Rather, accept it each day as a sacred gift necessary for good health.
5. Spend quality time in the kitchen and teach that cooking is a loving art not a drudgery. Emphasize both the beauty in food and that it is ultimately a source of health and vitality.
6. If a person has genuinely tried to enjoy a food, but the body seems to reject it, accept that as valid—at least for the time being.
7. Major on natural and raw foods and minor on the synthetic, artificial, and factory-processed food.
8. Refrain from purchasing food that is of no nutritional value.
9. Consider the use of supplemental vitamins to assure adequate supplies of nutrients for maximum health.

---

[1]Virginia and Norman Rohrer, *Junk Food: The Answer Book* (Old Tappan, New Jersey: Fleming H. Revell, 1983).

twenty-one

Exercise Is Not Spelled T-O-R-T-U-R-E

Now that you're getting thin, you will feel better physically. Now is the time to start exercising. When you were smaller, you probably played outside every day. Now that you are older, you don't like to do the same things you did when you were a small child. Maybe you even think you don't like exercise.

But physical fitness does not have to be horrible. God does not want you to be worn out and aching. Exercise can be fun if you start by choosing the exercise you like best.

Tim discovered he really liked soccer, but he didn't know he would like it so much until he tried it several times. Bonnie's friend, Betsy, took tennis lessons at the Y.

Bonnie never dreamed she would like to play tennis. "It looked too *hard*." But one day she went to Betsy's lesson with her and thought she might like to try it, too. Now Bonnie has been taking tennis lessons for over a month, and she just loves it. Bonnie always thought she was clumsy. In fact, her mother often joked about how clumsy she was. Bonnie found out she wasn't clumsy at all on the tennis court.

Terry was afraid of exercise. She thought that people would laugh at her if she participated in sports. Then one day her mother invited her to go along to an exercise class. There were people of all ages there and nobody made fun of her, so she felt as though she were part of the group. Now every week Terry looks forward to her exercise class. "In the beginning I could hardly keep up with everybody else," Terry said, "but now I do well and I have fun doing it."

Carey started jogging with his dad every morning. He walked and jogged in the beginning, but now he can jog a whole mile without stopping. He feels very happy with himself.

How to Get Started

If you want to eliminate your interest in exercise, just start an exercise program that is difficult and too demanding. That's what Sara did. Sara came home after the girls' basketball practice in tears. She was furious.

"I hate basketball!" Sara cried. "I feel *terrible*." Sara was angry because it was harder work than she had expected. Furthermore, she didn't have the vaguest idea how to play basketball and she felt like a fool out on the court. Sara learned from this experience. Instead of just trying the first thing she thought of, she first needed to ask herself what she *wanted* to try. Maybe at another time Sara will like girls' basketball, and maybe even become a star player. Right now was not the time for her to be placed in an important playing position she didn't want or like.

Instead, Sara thought about roller skating. Her youth group at church often went roller skating, but Sara had never joined them because she had been embarrassed. Now she decided to try it and she found out she loved roller skating. She became quite good at it, too.

Maybe swimming will be your favorite sport. Or perhaps you will find out you love softball or baseball. Maybe just walking or riding your bike will be the most fun. Give yourself time to learn what you like best.

Begin Slowly

You don't have to begin training for the next Olympic Games right away, you know. Any kind of exercise is better than no exercise. Don't worry about conquering the world today with your great athletic abilities. Slow and easy is the key. Be sure to have fun with whatever you do. If you don't want to be involved in team sports, why not get one of your parents or a brother or sister or someone else to play badminton or racquetball or to do some exercises on the floor with you? Here are some activities many young people on the *Slimming Down and Growing Up* program do on a regular basis:

Jogging	Golf
Bicycling	Softball
Swimming	Bowling
Skating	Walking
Handball/squash	Exercise class
Cross-country skiing	Downhill skiing
Basketball	Volleyball
Tennis	Badminton
Rowing	Wrestling
Hiking	Aerobic dancing
Tether ball	Clogging

Have you ever noticed how lazy and tired you feel when you just sit around all day? When you play and exercise you feel better. You have more energy. If you get involved in regular exercise you'll feel better and have more vim and vigor. But go at it easy. Have fun. Don't push yourself past your limit. The thing to remember is *have fun*.

Daily Power Time

Exercise can be fun. You can make sure it's fun if you choose what you *like* to do. Take Jesus with you when you exercise and play. It's even more fun to know He's there with you.

Scripture Verse for Today:

"*Commit your work to the Lord, then it will succeed*" (Proverbs 16:3).

My thoughts today: ________________________________

____

____

____

My special talk with God: ___________________________

What today's Scripture verse means to me:

To Say Out Loud

I will not be lazy anymore. I will enjoy exercising. I won't hurt myself by avoiding sports any longer. I will choose an activity that I think is fun and do it! Thank you, Jesus, for being with me.

twenty-two

Keeping an Exercise Record

You are ready now to start something new—keeping a daily exercise record. At the end of every day, write the activities you did during the day. Here is the chart you can use:

Exercise Activities

Time:	Activities:

If you walked to school, write it down on your chart. If you played ball in the schoolyard or took a P.E. class at school, write it down. Write the time if you can, also. At the end of the day you will see what times of day you exercised the most and what times of day you exercised the least.

Sara's exercise chart looked like this:

Time:	*Activities:*
8:00 AM	Ran without stopping one block to school bus.
11:00	P.E. class at school (played basketball).
3:00 PM	Walked home from bus stop.

When Sara looked at her chart, she realized that she hardly ever exercised after school or in the evening. She wanted to change that. The next day Sara's chart looked like this:

Time:	*Activities:*
8:00 AM	Ran one block without stopping to school bus.
11:00	P.E. class at school (played basketball).
3:00 PM	Walked home from bus stop.
3:30	Made a snowman outside in the yard with little brother.
7:00	Went roller skating with church youth group.

Sara made a real effort to add activities in the evenings and after school. Sara was becoming thinner and she wanted to be strong and healthy, too. Sometimes in the evenings she went swimming with her mother and younger brother to the indoor pool at the Y. Sometimes she went for a long walk in the snow with a friend. It was a wonderful surprise to discover she liked roller skating, and she made sure she went roller skating once a week.

Will I Always Have to Keep a Chart of What I Eat and How Much I Exercise?

Carey filled out his daily food chart and sighed. "Will I *always* have to do this?" he asked. "Will I *always* have to write down my food plan and exercise?" The answer is no. You, like Carey, are doing it now for a good purpose. You are on a weight-control program and while you are, you will want to fill in the charts and follow the lessons. But the program is only thirty days long. After this time you will have learned more about yourself and developed new habits. You won't have to keep charts forever because the *Slimming Down and Growing Up* program will become part of your life. Your new habits will be forever, even after you're done writing them down.

Questions to Answer

True or False:

_____ It's important to exercise in order to have energy and feel good.

_____ The secret of exercise is to find something you like to do.

_____ A little exercise is better than no exercise.

Answer:

1. My favorite exercise is: ______________________________

____

2. My favorite games are: ______________________________

____

3. Sports I like best to watch are: ______________________

____

4. Someday I would like to be able to (fill in an activity or sport): ______________________________________

____

5. An activity I am afraid to do is: ______________________

____

6. An activity I'm good at is: __________________________

____

Daily Power Time

Not exercising and staying fat is like being a slave to laziness and overweight, isn't it? Today's verse is about freedom and a new life complete with health, feeling good and doing activities that you enjoy and have fun at.

Scripture Verse for Today:

"Christ has made us free. Now make sure you stay free and don't get all tied up again in the chains of slavery. . ." (Galatians 5:1).

My thoughts today: ______________________________

____

____

My special talk with God:

What today's Scripture verse means to me:

To Say Out Loud

I am free to have fun doing things I like to do. Christ has set me free to exercise at my own pace and have fun doing it.

Just for Parents

Young people must develop skills of handling stress, anxiety, boredom, and depression in ways they can understand. Like adults, they can develop stress-related behaviors like intestinal disturbances, headaches, and irritability. One good way of handling stress is to become more physically active. And exercise can help hurry along a weight loss, too.

Many people falsely believe that it takes huge amounts of exercise to have any significant effect on weight loss, but it's not true. In order to take off one pound of weight, the average person has to burn up 3,500 calories. That means that if your child burns up only two hundred extra calories a day, 73,000 calories would go in a year. That would mean a loss of twenty pounds! And only twenty minutes of vigorous exercise is needed to take care of those two hundred calories.

Many obese people don't eat more than people of normal weight. A team of Harvard investigators discovered that the overweight schoolgirls they studied weren't consuming any more food than normal girls, but they were spending two-thirds less time in physical activity. It can make a difference!

Another common belief is that exercise increases the appetite. This is not true, either. According to the American Medical Association and the President's Council on Physical Fitness, moderate exercise will not stimulate the appetite.

Getting your youngster involved in a sport is probably the best way to encourage regular exercise. You may want to find an organized program for the sport in which your child shows an interest. However, stay clear of any highly competitive programs. You don't want your child to be refused on a team because of overweight or lack of skill. Your goal is not that your child win trophies or ribbons, but that he *participate*. Be sure your own expectations are not too high. Your child should not be expected to be an athlete.

It may help to start your child on an activity which he can do alone, like swimming or skating. Swimming uses all of the muscles of the body, and is a sport your child can do all of his life. You don't have to be on a team to ice skate or roller skate, either, and your child can improve at his own speed. He or she can also start by walking or slow jogging.

A two-person sport for you and your child will be helpful and fun. Be encouraging and have a good time. If you stress competition and skill, your child will feel intimidated and lose interest. Play to have fun.

Galatians 5:1 tells us that Christ has set us free. Remember that He has also set you free from anxiety and worry about your child. The One who liberated you from sin can free your child to be thin. You can relax and join your child in looking forward to success.

twenty-three

The Bible Story of Daniel's Special Diet

Even though he lived thousands of years ago, you and Daniel have a lot in common. He learned a special way of eating that was good for him, and he stuck to it even when it wasn't easy.

Chosen for the King's Service

Daniel was only about sixteen years old when an enemy, King Nebuchadnezzar, captured him and many other Jewish people and took them as slaves to his country of Babylon. There Daniel and some of his friends were chosen for three years of special training to be leaders in the new land. King Nebuchadnezzar picked out Daniel and the other boys because they were good looking and intelligent. They showed understanding and good sense, and they had the ability to serve.

Have you ever considered yourself in training for the king's personal service? The Lord Jesus is the King of Kings, and He has chosen you to serve Him. The Bible says, "*God the Father chose you long ago and knew you would become his children. And the Holy Spirit has been at work in your hearts, cleansing you with the blood of Jesus Christ and making you to please him*" (1 Peter 1:2).

Daniel Knew How to Obey

Even in this foreign land, Daniel decided to obey the rules God had given His people to live by. That meant Daniel refused the king's rich food, even though most of the other boys disobeyed God and ate it. The Bible says, "*Daniel resolved not to defile himself with the royal food and wine. . .*" (Daniel 1:8).

Defile means to make unclean. When we overeat or eat food that makes our bodies unhealthy, we defile ourselves. Daniel refused to defile himself with the king's food. He convinced the officers and the commander to allow him and his friends to eat vegetables and water for ten days. He claimed that at the end of ten days, he would be healthier and stronger than those who ate the fancier food.

Sure enough! Daniel and his friends were healthier, stronger, and felt better than all the other boys. So they were allowed to stay on their healthy diet.

Notice that Daniel *wanted* to keep on eating healthy foods. He did not complain. He didn't envy the others as they ate rich and heavy foods from the king's table because he wasn't interested in those fattening sweets.

Daniel knew how to obey because he loved God. King Nebuchadnezzar liked Daniel and his friends better than all the other young boys in the school.

When Daniel entered the king's service, he was consulted regarding important kingdom matters, and the king found Daniel and his friends ten times smarter and more faithful than all his other magicians and prophets. Daniel prospered because he *obeyed* God.

Will you say these words with us?

- I can obey the Lord.
- It is not hard to obey the Lord.
- Obeying the Lord is good for me.
- I will not defile my body.
- God is pleased when I obey. I can be like Daniel.

God is ready to help you. If you stumble He is not going to give up on you. God helped Daniel and honored him when he chose to eat his special diet. God may not be telling you to eat only the foods that Daniel did, but He has a food plan that is very special for you. He is teaching you to keep a daily eating and exercise plan. He wants you to have your Daily Power Time in His Word. As you do, He will bless you, just as He did Daniel.

Questions to Answer

1. Daniel was only about sixteen years old when he was taken away from his home to be trained for a foreign king's service. How do you suppose Daniel felt? ______________

____

2. Did Daniel drool over the king's rich food while he ate his plate of vegetables? ______________

3. Daniel and his friends were chosen because they were:

____ Intelligent ____ Sensible
____ Able to serve ____ Disobedient
____ Fat

4. 1 Peter 1:2 tells you that God the Father chose you long ago to become His child. The Holy Spirit has been at work in your heart, cleansing you so you can please God. How do you please God? ______________

____

Daily Power Time

Scripture Verse for Today:

"I am sure that God who began the good work within you will keep right on helping you grow in his grace until his task with you is finally finished. . ." (Philippians 1:6).

My thoughts today: ______________

____

____

____

My special talk with God: ______________

____

____

____

What today's Scripture verse means to me: ______________

____

____

____

Did you make your food plan for tomorrow? _____

Did you fill in your exercise chart? _____

To Say Out Loud

God chose me to be His child. The Holy Spirit is working in my heart so that I can please the Lord. I can please the Lord like Daniel by obeying God in my eating habits.

twenty-four

When You're Tempted to Cheat

God created you with His own hands. Did you know that? "*It is God himself who has made us what we are and given us new lives from Christ Jesus. . .*" (Ephesians 2:10). Therefore, you are a unique and special person—a very important person. You deserve to have good things, but those things do *not* include fattening and harmful foods.

It's important to God that you feel good. There may be lots of temptations to overeat, but God is with you to help. "*The Lord will work out his plans for my life. . .*" (Psalm 138:8). You are going to stick with your program no matter how long it takes.

Here are some more helps for you when you are tempted to overeat:

1. *Enjoy your food.* Eating is not a sin. Enjoy the food God gives you to eat. We thank the Lord for our daily bread because He wants us to eat to be strong and healthy.
2. *Don't cut out the foods you like.* Count them on your daily food plan. Don't starve yourself.
3. *Measure your food.* Have fun when you measure your food. See if you can guess how much a half cup or a quarter of a cup is when you serve yourself food.
4. *When you eat in a restaurant, before you get there, think about what you'll eat.* Sometimes when you look at a menu, there are so many things to choose from that all of it looks

good. Remember you are a slimming down kid at home *and* at the restaurant.

5. *Don't be afraid to ask questions.* When you're at a restaurant, you can ask if a certain dish is rich and fattening. Some dishes will be new to you, so don't be afraid to ask what's in them.
6. *Ask your parents to keep plenty of fresh cut-up vegetables and fruit in the refrigerator for you to nibble on.* You could even cut up some vegetables and fruit for yourself and keep them in the refrigerator for those times when you want a snack.
7. *Drink a glass of water when you feel hungry.* You won't feel so hungry, and besides, your body needs water.
8. *Tell your friends and family that you're getting thin.* You're slimming down now and you no longer eat the way you used to.
9. *When you bring your lunch to school, make it healthy.* A sandwich of meat, on whole-wheat bread, fruit and a healthy treat is a good lunch.
10. *Go back and repeat your favorite Slimming Down and Growing Up lessons.* You may repeat the lessons in this book as many times as you want to. They are always there to help you.
11. *Include someone else.* If you do your *Slimming Down and Growing Up* program with someone else, you will have a partner who is working toward the same goal as you are. Maybe you can start a group with kids who want to get thin. If there are no kids in your area, you can do it all by yourself because you have everything you need.

Sometimes you will feel tempted, but it won't last. After you have been on the *Slimming Down and Growing Up* program for thirty days, you will have developed new habits that will last. Exercise and eating better foods are going to make a wonderful difference in your life.

Go at an Easy Pace

Don't allow yourself to be discouraged. Be good to yourself and when you exercise tell yourself, "This makes me feel good, too." Galatians 6:9 says, "*Let us not get tired of doing what is right, for after a while we will reap a harvest of blessing if we don't get discouraged and give up.*"

Tell yourself, "*I won't give up. I've been terrific so far and I won't lose heart even when I'm tempted. I won't get weary or tired of my new way of eating now. I will go at a slow and easy pace. I will tell myself, 'Good for me,' and I will thank the Lord.*"

Questions to Answer

1. When you are invited to go out to a restaurant and eat, what should you do? ______________________

____

2. What are some good snack foods to keep in the refrigerator? ______________________________

____

____

3. When you are tempted to overeat, what Bible verse is a good one to remember? ______________________

____

4. "*Let us not get tired of doing what is* ________, *for after a while we will reap a harvest of* ____________ *if we don't get discouraged and* ________________" (Galatians 6:9).

Daily Power Time

Scripture Verse for Today:

"*But remember this—the wrong desires that come into your life aren't anything new and different. Many others have faced exactly the same problems before you. And no temptation is irresistible. You can trust God to keep the temptation from becoming so strong that you can't stand up against it, for he has promised this and will do what he says. He will show you how to escape temptation's power so that you can bear up patiently against it*" (1 Corinthians 10:13).

My thoughts today: ______________________________

____

____

____

My special talk with God: ________________________

____

____

____

What today's Scripture verse means to me: __________

____

____

____

To Say Out Loud

God helps me be strong when I am tempted to do wrong. He promises that He will show me how to escape temptation. I can succeed and not get weary on my *Slimming Down and Growing Up* program no matter how long it takes to reach my goal. I am a winner!

Just for Parents

Daniel's diet was beautifully balanced with vitamins, minerals and protein. It must have included combinations of such vegetables as cabbage, onions, celery, cucumbers, lettuce, greens, tomatoes, potatoes, cheese, lentils and various beans. Going on Daniel's vegetable and water diet would take nutritional counsel. Before considering such a diet, be sure that all the necessary vitamins, minerals and protein are included. An average person needs at least forty to sixty grams of protein a day. We wrote about Daniel, not to encourage his diet, but to encourage your child to obey God as Daniel did.

Daniel chose not to defile himself with ungodly food. Your child needs help and strength from the Lord to turn away from the same foods Daniel refused. "*Those who let themselves be controlled by their lower natures live only to please themselves, but those who follow after the Holy Spirit find themselves doing the things that please God*" (Romans 8:5).

Our worldly minds, our selfishness, and our flesh sometimes become uncontrolled, but we can learn control. Getting control of the flesh means to become dominated by the influence and power of the Holy Spirit.

Food is not meant to tempt and tantilize you or your child. Food is meant to bless and strengthen you. It is meant to satisfy bodily needs for nourishment. Stuffing ourselves with fattening junk never satisfies. Will you remind your child about junk food? Perhaps today's version of Nebuchadnezzar's rich food goes by the name of "The Whopper" or "Big Mac."

Daniel had to learn how to obey God in his eating. We believe your child can do the same.

twenty-five

Doing What You Want Most of All

Maybe there was a time when you craved a cream-filled doughnut or some other rich, fattening food. But you are changing. You now have a different desire—to be thin, and please the Lord by what you eat. You are seeing God fulfill your new desire and give you much more besides, like more happiness, better health, and more energy. He's helping you do what you want most of all, because what you want is what He wants, too.

The Bible says, *"Be delighted with the Lord. Then he will give you all your heart's desires"* (Psalm 37:4). When you choose to obey God by eating His way, you are delighting in Him. He promises in return that He will give you what you want most.

What else do you really want? What are the desires of your heart? Many younger people on the *Slimming Down and Growing Up* plan find it helps to write them down, and you may want to, too. Then you can write down ideas of ways to cooperate with the Lord so He can give you those desires.

Connie wrote down her desires and actions this way:

Desire: I desire to be thin and not fat anymore.

Action: I will cooperate with the Lord by being faithful to my *Slimming Down and Growing Up* program. I will keep my daily food plan. I will keep my exercise sheet every day. I will have my Daily Power Time. I will say no to stuffing myself.

Desire: I desire to be on the girls' basketball team.

Action: I will cooperate with the Lord by practicing basketball and by watching the game. I will not give up or quit.

Don't you think Connie's Desire-Action Sheet is a good one? The actions she chose will help her move toward what she wants most. She's cooperating with the Lord, and she can expect Him to help her.

Terry Gets an Answer

Terry wasn't sure what her desires were. She thought and thought, but it took a long time to decide what to write. Finally she put down, "I desire to be Terry and the best Terry I can be." Then she had to stop and think again to decide what action might help her become what she wanted. One day Terry realized how often she heard herself complaining.

She knew that griping and complaining didn't please the Lord, and instead of making her the best she could be, they only made her negative and more unhappy. She wrote as her Action, "I will stop complaining. I will praise the Lord instead."

Tim Makes a Clearer Goal

Someone asked Tim, "What do you want most of all?" Before Tim started the *Slimming Down and Growing Up* program, he didn't know what he wanted to do. He only knew he was lonely and unhappy. He felt inferior to the boys in his class who were good in sports, but he could never play with them because he felt he was too fat. Playing sports and being with the other kids was what he wanted most, but instead of admitting and going after what he wanted, he went home to eat instead. Sweets and heavy breads and pastries only made Tim fatter and lonelier and farther away from fulfilling his real desires.

After Tim asked the Lord to help him grow thin, Tim could say, "I want to be happy and doing what I like to do." The Lord helped Tim find actions that fit his desires. Now he's playing soccer, and he's going to his church youth group instead of staying home alone.

What Do You Want Most?

Think about what matters to you. Your desires can work together with your actions to produce results. If your desire is to be able to run a mile without stopping, write it down. Decide what action you can take to begin cooperating with God to see that desire come true.

As you think about what you want, will you pray this prayer?

> Dear Lord Jesus, I'm going to give you my desires, and act like you are the leader of my life. I'm going to act like I am your child by obeying you. In Jesus' name, Amen.

Questions to Answer

1. Psalm 37:4 tells us we should delight in Someone. Complete the verse: "Be delighted with ________________. Then _______ will give you all your heart's desires."
2. What is your desire? ______________________________
3. What action can you take to cooperate with the Lord to fulfill your desire? ______________________________

____

Daily Power Time

Scripture Verse for Today:

"*Be delighted with the Lord. Then he will give you all your heart's desires*" (Psalm 37:4).

My thoughts today: ______________________________

____

____

____

My special talk with God: ______________________________

____

What today's Scripture verse means to me:

To Say Out Loud

The Lord will answer my prayer. He will grant me my desires because I delight myself in Him.

twenty-six

You're Having Fun Now

When Sara saw all the food on the table at her school's Valentine Day party, she swallowed in dismay. There was cake, candy, plates of heart-shaped cookies and sugary punch. That morning she had thought about the party and had written "two cookies" on her daily food plan. Now she faced all those goodies in front of her. The other boys and girls were filling their paper plates. Sara was tempted to forget she was slimming down and gobble up everything in sight.

Sara did not give in. She ate exactly two cookies. When she went home she had a good, healthy dinner and she felt full and happy. Sara gave herself a reward when she didn't give in. She made herself feel good by *not* overeating.

If Sara had eaten cake, cookies, candy and had punch besides, she would not have been doing *good* for herself. She would have been hurting herself and she would have felt bad afterward. But Sara rewarded herself when she ate with control.

More Rewards

A reward is something that is good for you and makes you feel good. Sara felt good when she said no to overeating. A reward is when you can say "Good for me" to yourself. Are you rewarding yourself the right way?

Last summer Jamie received a reward she had dreamed of ever since she was a little girl. When she was younger she had watched the water-skiers on the lake and wished she could water-ski, too. "It looked like so much fun," she said. "But I was clumsy and uncoordinated and couldn't get up on the skis. I stopped trying and wishing because it was embarrassing and awful. I felt big and fat." Every year when Jamie vacationed at the lake with her family, she watched other vacationers having fun in the water. "I just watched because I was afraid to try anything new. The other kids could dive and race in the water, but I could only play at it. It made me mad.

"My reward for staying on my *Slimming Down and Growing Up* program came in a wonderful way," Jamie beamed. Last summer she water-skied for the first time. After many tries she finally rose up on the skis and stayed up. Around the lake she went with her feet steady on the skis, her body sure and strong. Jamie never felt happier than that first time when she soared over the water, weaving back and forth across the waves as the boat ahead zoomed forward. "It was like I was flying," Jamie said. "Being able to water-ski was the greatest reward possible."

Everybody likes rewards. It's fun to be rewarded after working hard or doing a job well. Sometimes other people reward us, like when we win a trophy or earn extra money for doing extra chores. But you can reward *yourself* when you do something well.

Getting thinner and stronger is a reward for staying on your *Slimming Down and Growing Up* program. You deserve to be rewarded every day as you keep up the good work. Tell yourself, "Good for me, I did well again today!"

The Many Kinds of Rewards

Can you add some rewards to the list you made in Chapter Nine? Old rewards may have been money, presents, food, or a medal. What new kinds of rewards have you allowed yourself? Look at the things you like to *do* as a reward. Carey said one of his favorite things to do is work on his model airplane. Bonnie likes taking pictures with her camera. Terry likes ceramic painting.

Every week you should do something special as a reward for doing well on the *Slimming Down and Growing Up* program. In addition to the list on page 64, here are some more special rewards other *Slimming Down and Growing Up* young people have chosen:

- Go to a special movie.
- Go to a ballgame.
- Play a game with a parent.
- Make a long distance call to a special friend or relative.
- Go to work with a parent.
- Get out of doing dishes for one day.
- Go to the zoo.
- Go to the theater.
- Stay up one hour later.
- Have a friend spend the night.
- Read a favorite book.
- Take a bubble bath.
- Go water-skiing.

These are all *doing* rewards. List some of your own favorite *doing* rewards.

God is pleased when you trust Him and work hard at accomplishing your goal. He likes to reward you. He tells you, "Well done, good and faithful servant. . . ." You can reward yourself the same way, because you're working hard toward your goal. God is with you and you are doing a good job.

A Reminder

Maybe when you were younger you thought of sweets or dessert as a reward. Now you know that rewards are not what you eat, but what you *do*.

You can feel good about yourself—the Lord feels good about you! When you obey Him by reading His Word and following His directions, you feel good. *Your reward is feeling good*. Jesus is the Lord of your life and the Lord of your eating habits. You are safe from making the old mistakes again and again.

Questions to Answer

Check One:

1. A reward is: something that makes you feel good about

yourself _____; something that makes you rich _____.

2. You can reward yourself by: doing something that's fun to do _____; having something rich and fattening to eat _____.

3. Name three "doing" rewards: ______________________, ______________________, ______________________.

4. How does the Lord reward you? ______________________
____

5. Did you exercise today? __________

Daily Power Time

Scripture Verse for Today:

"*For the mountains may depart and the hills disappear, but my kindness shall not leave you*" (Isaiah 54:10).

My thoughts today: ______________________________
____
____
____

My special talk with God: __________________________
____
____
____

What today's Scripture verse means to me: ___________
____
____
____

To Say Out Loud

The Lord rewards me. He helps me to choose rewards that are good for me. I do not reward myself by eating, but by doing something fun and something that makes me feel good.

Just for Parents

Psalm 37:4 tells us that if we take delight in God, He will give us our heart's desire. A desire is a longing and wanting. A child may call it a wish. When our desires are in the right place—that is, when we desire to *please* the Lord—our lives are in good order.

Delight means a "high degree of pleasure or enjoyment; joy, great pleasure and satisfaction." Your child may desire to please the Lord, but is there delight in it? The Lord is not a cruel master. He isn't standing over your child with a stick, ready to swat him for eating wrongly. If your child gets this impression of God, he may outwardly obey Him but inwardly harbor resentment.

Your son or daughter is not deprived because of eating the right foods. God *gives*. He restores His children, lifts us up to new heights, builds and strengthens us. Satan destroys, lies, and deceives, often about food.

Talk with your child about the commercials on radio and television, and in magazines. Are they realistic? Advertisements always depict eating as one of the most joyous and exuberant events in life. A simple hamburger or can of soda is made to look like a king's feast, or a monument of art and ecstasy. But no matter how they make it look, a candy bar simply is not a triumph of social, intellectual and gastronomic bliss.

Be sure your child knows the people in these commercials are actors, and that writers made up the words they speak. They are not real. If those actors actually ate all the fattening foods they say they do in commercials, they'd be too fat to get a job on television!

As your child learns to separate fantasy from reality, his healthy diet of good foods will begin to look better to him, and he'll be freer to genuinely delight in doing God's will.

Be sure to encourage your youngster's exercise and play today. Observe if he is sleeping too much, or sitting in front of the television too long. In fact, why don't you put down this book right now and suggest you take a walk together? It may prove to be a delight to you both.

twenty-seven

Pushing Your Own Buttons

Do you know what self-control is? Jill answered the question like this. "Self-control is like last night when I said no to two helpings of mashed potatoes and gravy and had only one helping instead. Self-control is when I turned down the cherry pie and chose strawberries instead."

Making Your Own Decisions

"Self-control is pushing your own buttons," Tim said. That's a good way of saying it's making your own decisions. Jill pushed the self-control button inside her mind and made two good decisions when she chose not to overeat.

If you were flying in an airplane and you wanted to land, you'd have to know which buttons to push, wouldn't you? And if you are at the dinner table with lots of food in front of you, you have to know which buttons to push, too.

Buttons are decisions. You *decide*, "No, I didn't plan for two helpings. I won't have them." You *decide* to have red, juicy strawberries instead of heavy cherry pie. That's self-control. It's pushing your own decision control buttons.

You Have Self-Control

Sometimes you may not feel like you have any self-control because you didn't refuse two helpings of dessert. But you may have more self-control than you think you do. Bonnie and Betsy found they did.

Bonnie sighed and looked at her friend, Betsy, enviously. "Betsy, you have so much self-control. You can say no to foods you know are not good for you."

"But you have self-control, too, Bonnie," Betsy answered her. "You keep your room clean, don't you?"

Bonnie thought a minute. She did keep her room clean. Even if she didn't always feel like it, she put away her clothes and made her bed. That *did* take some self-control, didn't it?

"We're showing self-control a lot of ways," Bonnie said. "We do our *Slimming Down and Growing Up* lessons every day, don't we? And we write our daily food and exercise plans."

"Yes, and I'm going for walks every day," Betsy reminded her, "and you're exercising more than you ever have before."

It was wrong to say they had no self-control. Both girls were showing self-control in many parts of their lives. When you think you don't have self-control, remember the times when you had it in the past.

Tim said, "I push my self-control button when I do my homework. I don't always want to do homework when there are more fun things to do, but I push my self-control button anyhow. See? I have self-control."

Sara said, "I have self-control, too. Today I did the dishes right away when my mom told me to. I didn't want to, but I did."

Here are some ways you probably show self-control:

- *You get up on time in the morning*. You control your urge to go on sleeping.
- *You get to school on time*. You don't waste time getting ready for school.
- *You answer the phone when it rings*. Sometimes you may be busy, but you still answer the phone. Even if you're sleeping, you get up to answer the phone.
- *You take a bath or shower regularly*. You take responsibility to keep yourself clean.
- *You brush your teeth*. Even though it's easy to forget, you remember to brush.

And there are probably many other ways. Do you get your homework in on time? Do you fold your clothes in your drawer, or hang them in the closet? Do you make your bed? Each time you do, you prove you *do* have self-control. Since you do, you can expect your self-control to grow, too, as you face tempting foods.

Self-control is:

- Something God wants you to have.
- Pushing your own buttons so you do what you know God wants you to do (like getting out of bed in the morning when the alarm clock rings).
- Doing something that's good for you when you don't want to do it.
- Doing something that's hard to do.
- Making decisions.

Pat Yourself on the Back

Because you are God's child, He wants many good things for you. Some of those things are listed in Galatians 5:22–23. They're called the "fruit," or the results, that the Holy Spirit produces as He lives in your life. They are love, joy, peace, patience, kindness, goodness, faithfulness, gentleness, and *self-control.* You can have self-control because God wants you to. When you ask God for self-control, He helps you.

Self-control is more than pushing your "No" button. It's pushing your "Yes" button, too. Self-control means to say *yes* to health and feeling good. It means saying *yes* to trusting God instead of worrying.

When you push your self-control button, tell yourself, "Good for me!" Be happy when you show self-control, and pat yourself on the back. Every time you refuse dessert, smile and say, "I pushed my self-control button! I'm terrific!"

A Prayer for You

Dear Jesus, thank you for my self-control. Thank you that I am learning to push my self-control buttons in the area of eating. Thank you for helping me. In Jesus' name, Amen.

Questions to Answer

1. Which foods especially tempt you to lose self-control? List those foods which have been hard for you to say no to in the past:

____________________ ____________________

____________________ ____________________

____________________ ____________________

____________________ ____________________

True or False:

____ Self-control is eating whatever you want when you feel like it.
____ You show self-control when you get to school on time.
____ You show self-control when you lie on the sofa and watch TV instead of washing the dishes like your mother asked.
____ Self-control is making a decision.

Complete the following:

1. Self-control is knowing how to say no and knowing how to say ____.

2. The fruit of the Holy Spirit in Galatians 5:22–23 are: love, joy, peace, _____, _____, _____, _____, _____, _____.

3. What are some ways you show self-control every day?

____

____

____

____

4. How did you show self-control today at your meals?

____

____

Daily Power Time

After David killed Goliath, he became a favorite with the king, but it didn't last long. David had many troubles in his life and he prayed to the Lord to help him. David knew that he couldn't win any battles or overcome any struggles without the help of the Lord. He knew his own strength was not enough.

The Bible tells us it's O.K. to be weak, because then God can show us how strong He is.

Scripture Verse for Today:

"*Let the weak be strong*" (Joel 3:10).

My thoughts today: ____________________

____

____

____

My special talk with God: ____________________

____

____

____

What today's Scripture verse means to me: ____________________

____

____

____

To Say Out Loud

I can say I'm strong because I belong to God. He is my strength. I have self-control because God helps me.

twenty-eight

Emergency! What to Do If You Fail

What happens when you overeat one day and forget all about your *Slimming Down and Growing Up* plan? How about if you refuse to exercise and spend the day just sitting in front of the TV? Should you give up and head for the nearest doughnut shop?

Never!

You may have goofed, but God is still with you. Confess to the Lord that you have failed. Ask for His forgiveness and then go on. God will help you start over again. If you sneaked some food, or if you cheated, or if you told yourself a lie, *God still forgives.* He says, "*If we confess our sins to him, he can be depended on to forgive us and to cleanse us from every wrong*" (1 John 1:9). And He promises, "*I have blotted out your sins; they are gone like morning mist at noon! Oh, return to me, for I have paid the price to set you free*" (Isaiah 44:22).

Go on! Return to your program and keep going. Don't tell yourself to wait until tomorrow. Start now. Don't skip meals to try to make up for what you overeat.

Nobody Is Hopeless

If you feel bad about overeating, remember that you are not hopeless. God says, "*Fear not, for I am with you. Do not be dismayed. I am your God. I will strengthen you; I will help you; I will uphold you with my victorious right hand*" (Isaiah 41:10).

Even if you didn't do your lesson yesterday, you can do it today. Even if you don't want to do your Daily Power Time, you can start over. When you complete your *Slimming Down and Growing Up* program, you will have begun a lifelong way of eating. Even if learning those new habits takes longer than thirty days, don't get discouraged and quit.

You're learning how to eat. You may want to lose weight faster than it wants to get lost. If you are kind to yourself, you will give yourself another chance.

Sometimes people who are overweight are very hard on themselves. They don't think that they are very good people. Tim didn't think he was a good person. Neither did the other young people we wrote about in this book. Bonnie didn't like herself; Jill didn't like herself; Connie was unhappy about herself, and so were Terry, Jamie and Sara. Each one of them had to learn that it's O.K. not to be perfect. Nobody is hopeless.

Liking Yourself

It's easy to forget how well you're doing when you do something you don't like. Jamie thought she was a total failure because she overate one day. She didn't look at all the days when she had self-control. She couldn't think of rewarding herself now because she felt so terrible.

Getting thin takes time. If you will tell yourself, "I like me. I'm O.K.," you will feel good about yourself. You are a special person. Because you're so special, you deserve good things, and you deserve to be patient with yourself.

It will only take longer for you to get back on the right track if you feel bad and say bad things about yourself or others. Maybe you're mad at your mother. Maybe you're mad at us. Have you heard yourself say, "This whole program is a dumb idea"? Maybe you're mad at your friends who can eat anything they want. If you blame your overeating on someone else, you will only take longer to get going again. Blame your overeating on the fact that you made a mistake, period. It's O.K. to make a mistake. Jesus is there with you to pick you up again and help you start all over.

You're a Winner!

Winners always return to the Lord when they've made a mistake and start over again. You are not a loser. You've come this far and you're going to go on.

Don't Give Up!

- No matter how slow the going seems, *don't give up.*
- Even if you gain weight, *don't give up.*
- Even if you don't feel like going on, *don't give up.*
- Even if you're tired of *Slimming Down and Growing Up, don't give up.*
- Even if you feel you're all alone, *don't give up.*
- Whatever you do, wherever you are, *don't give up.*

A Prayer to Pray

Dear Lord, thank you for giving me the courage not to give up. Thank you for forgiving me. Thank you for showing me I'm O.K., no matter what. Thank you for helping me go on and not stop now. In Jesus' name, Amen.

Questions to Answer

Complete:

1. *"Fear not, for I am ______ ______. Do not be dismayed. I am ______ ______. I will __________ you; I will ______ you; I will ____________ you with my victorious right hand"* (Isaiah 41:10).

Daily Power Time

Scripture Verse for Today:

"If we confess our sins to him, he can be depended on to forgive us and to cleanse us from every wrong" (1 John 1:9).

My thoughts today: ______________________________

____

My special talk with God:

What today's Scripture verse means to me:

To Say Out Loud

I like myself. I am not giving up. I am a winner. God forgives me and helps me now and always will.

Just for Parents

Have you ever thanked God for the privilege of learning self-control? Self-control is a priceless jewel, and the Lord may be using this struggle against overweight to give this jewel to your child—or to you. "*It was good for me to be afflicted, so that I might learn your decrees*" (Psalm 119:71, NIV).

One mother said, "I never dreamed there would be anything good about being fat, but struggling against those pounds has brought me to the point in my life where I am willing to learn about God and His ways. It was good for me that I gained weight, and had to fight to lose it, so that I can become a far more powerful Christian than I otherwise would have chosen to be."

Another woman paraphrased Psalm 119:71 this way, "Because I am fat, I am now learning about self-control. . . . It is good for me that I have been afflicted with fat in order that I can reach such a wonderful nose-to-nose position with God."[1]

If you are excited about good food, your child will be, too. A "delightful" verse to remember is Psalm 119:16, "*I will delight in your decrees. . . .*" If you delight in drinking a glass of fruit juice when everyone else is eating chocolate pie, your child will see your example and not feel so weird when he says no to fattening food. If you delight in serving lean meat, broiled chicken, fish, fresh vegetables and fruits, whole-grains and fresh eggs and cheeses, your child will be blessed with a good example to follow.

Dear Parent, while you encourage your child, be sure to include a "Good for me!" We know it is hard work to reprogram wrong eating habits. We salute you and praise God for you. Give yourself a big pat on the back.

---

[1]Marie Chapian and Neva Coyle, *Free To Be Thin* (Minneapolis: Bethany House Publishers, 1979), p. 119.

twenty-nine

Eating a Daily Feast

You may not become a weight lifter, or a track star, or a football hero, but we can all be heroes in God's eyes. We can all be mighty members of God's army.

You can have faith like David. As you sit down to eat, you can say as David did to his enemy Goliath, "Food, I come to you in the name of the Lord." You can tell the candy store and the pizza place and the ice cream shop: "The battle is the Lord's. The Lord who saved me from overeating and stuffing myself will go on saving me from overeating and stuffing myself."

But David didn't pray just when he faced trouble. He talked to the Lord often. He had regular "special talks with God," just like you do. If you read the book of Psalms in the Bible, you'll see some of the songs and prayers David wrote to the Lord in his Daily Power Time.

Even after you've finished your thirty-day *Slimming Down and Growing Up* program, you will still want to keep on with your Daily Power Time, and feast on the Word of God. As you read God's Word and pray, God will help you with many other parts of your life besides just your eating.

Connie Gets Help in School

Connie's parents had considered having her repeat sixth grade because her grades had been so poor. The last thing Connie wanted was to be held back, so she prayed for the Lord's help.

In her Daily Power Time one morning, she thought about the story of David killing Goliath. David stood up against his enemy in the name of the Lord, and he won the battle. Connie felt repeating sixth grade was her enemy, so she decided to do what David had done.

"I will not only eat in the name of the Lord," Connie said. "I will do my schoolwork in the name of the Lord, too." Connie asked the Lord to help her understand her schoolwork. She could do this because she knew and believed His Word. God answered her prayers and she did not get held back. Also, this year she is making good grades.

"The Lord helped me," she smiles. "I really have to thank Him."

When Connie studied the Word of God, her mind opened up to understand His ways. She learned to love His Word and her daily times with the Lord. Then when Connie did her schoolwork, she discovered that learning was easier.

God said, "*Call to me and I will answer you and tell you great and unsearchable things you do not know*" (Jeremiah 33:3, NIV). God can teach you what you need to know about Him as you continue to meet with Him every day.

Here are some ideas to help make your Daily Power Time an energy-producing feast you can enjoy all your life:

1. Be sure your Bible is written in language you can understand. *The Living Bible* is a favorite among young people because it is written in everyday language. Other translations you might like are the *New International Version* and the *Amplified Version*.

2. After you've finished your thirty-day program in this book, begin your Bible reading in the New Testament. The New Testament starts with the life of Jesus, and every day you'll learn new things about Him and how He can help you. The first four books of the New Testament (Matthew, Mark, Luke and John) all talk about Jesus' life. Some kids like to read John's book first before the other three because it's easier to understand.

3. You can read some verses, or even a chapter of the Bible every day, and then choose one of the verses to think about especially that day, and to repeat out loud to yourself.

4. Record your Daily Power Time in your special notebook. Every day write down the place in the Scripture you read that day. Record your thoughts, your special talk with God, and what today's Scripture meant to you, just as you have been doing in this book. If you're not as thin yet as you want to be, this notebook can become a great place to write your daily food plan and exercise record, too, until your goal is reached.

5. Reading your favorite Bible characters is another fun way to learn from the Bible. You might want to take one Bible character a week, and read part of their story each day. When you get ready to write "My Thoughts Today," you can put down some of the ways you'd like to be like that person. Your parents or minister can help you find the stories in the Bible, if you need them to.

6. Share what God is showing you during your Daily Power Time with somebody else.

Daily Power Time

Scripture Verse for Today:

"Call to me and I will answer you and tell you great and unsearchable things you do not know" (Jeremiah 33:3, NIV).

My thoughts today: ______________________________

____

____

____

My special talk with God: __________________________

____

____

____

What today's Scripture verse means to me: ______________

____

____

____

To Say Out Loud

I am glad God answers my prayers and that I can trust Him, even when I'm not sure I can trust myself. He is always there ready to help.

thirty

Look at You Now!

Now that you are at the very end of your *Slimming Down and Growing Up* program, you have tasted victory and you have worked hard. Here are some of the things that caused you to overeat in the first place and that you now know how to fight:

Angry feelings. Sara said, "Before I was a slimming down kid, I was angry all the time and I overate. Now I feel good about myself. I have almost reached my goal. I don't get angry as much anymore. Once when I got angry around the fourteenth lesson in this book, I wanted to overeat. I realized being angry and overeating went together. Now I tell myself I will not overeat if I get angry."

Being bored. When you feel bored and want to eat, remember that is how you got fat. Now if you are bored, you go for a run, a walk, call somebody, do something fun, and stay away from the refrigerator.

Feeling lonely. When Jill moved away from the home she loved, she felt lonely. She overate to make the feelings of loneliness go away, but it didn't work. Now when you feel lonely, you won't head for the kitchen or the candy store. You head for new ideas on how to make new friends. There are many friends just waiting to meet you and know you. All you have to do is be friendly and get out of the kitchen.

Here are some final words of strength for you. Remember them and you will have mastery over bad habits.

1. *Don't* eat while watching TV.
2. *Don't* eat while studying or doing homework. (Wait until you take a little break and then have a snack or a glass of water.)
3. *Don't* eat while reading. Be good to yourself. Enjoy your book without getting fat.
4. *Don't* eat while walking somewhere or when riding in the car. (These times are not for eating. They are for going somewhere and noticing the things around you. Eat your three meals and three snacks only.)
5. *Don't* eat while setting the table or helping in the kitchen. (Wait until you sit down at the table. You will be glad you did.)
6. *Don't* eat while cleaning up after a meal. (When you are clearing the dishes or helping to clean the kitchen, don't eat the leftovers. You are not a garbage disposal. You are a precious child of God.)
7. *Don't* eat more when you are by yourself. (Be good to yourself at all times. When you are with others, or by yourself you are a free-to-be-thin kid. You are doing well! Congratulate yourself and stop eating in secret.)
8. *Don't* get out of bed in the middle of the night to eat. (Your stomach deserves a good night's sleep.)
9. *Don't* eat more at night than during the day. (Do something fun instead of eating. Remember to do your exercise activity. Have fun.)
10. *Don't* skip breakfast. (Breakfast is energy time. You need your morning energy.)

Questions to Answer

1. Name three emotions that usually trigger overeating:

   a. ____________________

   b. ____________________

   c. ____________________

2. Name two don'ts:

a. ____________________

b. ____________________

3. How has your *Slimming Down and Growing Up* program affected your family? ____________________

____

____

4. Now that you are at the last day of your *Slimming Down and Growing Up* program, name one change in your life that is the most special to you: ____________________

____

____

Daily Power Time

Scripture Verse for Today:

"*Because the Lord is my Shepherd, I have everything I need!*" (Psalm 23:1).

With the Lord as your Shepherd, you have successfully completed thirty days on your *Slimming Down and Growing Up* program. We congratulate you and thank God for you. How wonderful you must feel now that you have experienced a new way of eating with the Lord as your helper.

My thoughts today: ____________________

____

____

____

My special talk with God: ____________________

____

____

____

What today's Scripture verse means to me: ______________

____

____

____

To Say Out Loud

I'll never go back to being fat and unhappy because the Lord is my Shepherd and I now have everything I need. I can eat healthy now. I can exercise now and feel good. My new habits will last forever because the Lord helps me and loves me.

thirty-one

A Note from Neva, Just for Parents . . . .

Whenever I see an overweight child, my heart is touched with compassion, understanding, and also my own memories. It is because of this tenderness born out of my own experience that I have wanted this book written.

I do not expect, nor should you, that when your child has finished with this project that his or her weight problem will be solved. Your child, will, however, have been given some effective tools to battle and overcome this problem.

There will be days when you will think that none of this effort has done any good, but it has. The training that this study has given will not leave your child even as he or she grows into adulthood.

Be a support, not a judge or spy. Be loving and accepting along with being firm. Let your child know how much you love him or her and how much you admire the effort put forth during his study and also acknowledge the sacrifice with which your child is faced.

Most of all, pray for your child. Do not ever say, "What can I do for my child, except just pray?" Prayer is essential and your child needs it. During weight loss times is when God has done the most changing in my attitudes and I have grown the deepest spiritually when I have used these times of weight control challenge to get closer to Jesus Christ.

I praise God for loving, caring parents who cared enough to purchase this book for their child.

Blessings on you,
Because of Jesus,

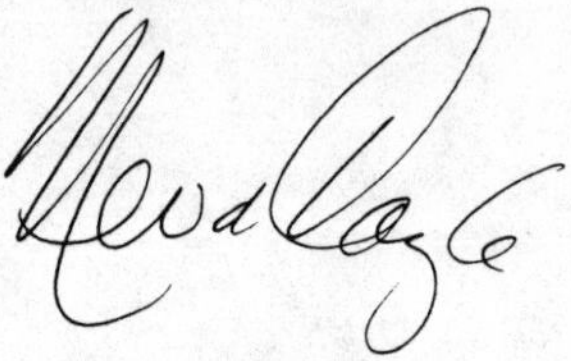

Neva Coyle

Appendix: National Research Council's Recommended Daily Caloric Allowances

	Age	Weight		Height		Calories
		*(kg)	(lbs.)	**(cm)	(in.)	
Children	7–10	30	66	135	54	2,400
Males	11–14	44	97	158	63	2,800
Males	15–18	61	134	172	69	3,000
Females	11–14	44	97	155	62	2,400
Females	15–18	54	119	162	65	2,100